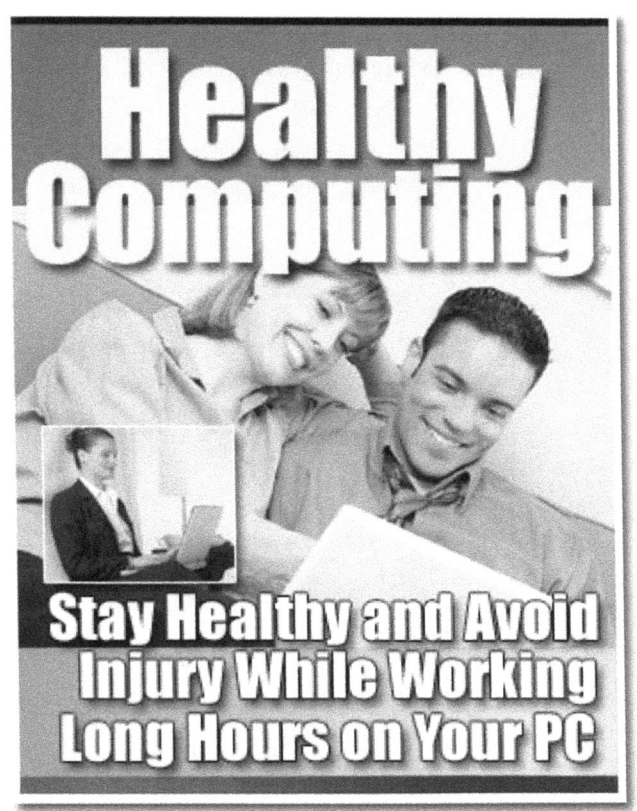

Table of Contents

Introduction

There is no other device that changed our lives like computers.

The growth of computers and related technologies has been so unprecedented that, it has found a place in every aspect of human life. Be it for fun, relaxation or money, people use this device widely so much that, it's found in almost every establishment. Philosophically, everything in life comes with a clause. It's same with the so-called magic device, 'computer'. There has been a lot of discussion in the media about the side effects of using computers for a long time. After revolutionizing the world with its multitude of uses, the health hazards of long time computer usage became a real revelation for the millions of computer users. It all started in the 80's and as years passed, more studies revealed many astonishing facts. The most common ailments related to computer usage are vision defects and wrist injuries. According to American optometric association, 12 million Americans visit eye doctors due to computer related problems. Though these facts can be quite frightening, you need not panic as a little care can make you devoid of these even if you are a regular computer user.

Computers are used by millions of people every day around the world. And each of them will have their own styles of working and hence there cannot be a single correct arrangement of components that will work well with everyone. A transcriptionist may find things easier if the arrangement enables her fast and accurate typing while a graphic artist may like to have his work station done in a way that foster his thinking. Try imagining your workstation as you go through each section and visualize if you can identify where you have to improve on your posture, placement of system components and the workstation. This is an e-guide on tips and ticks to minimize or eradicate your identified stress and strain while using your computer and how to stay healthy though you have to work on your computer all day and thus enables you to design your own workstation.

These days, computers have become so inevitable part of our lives that we need to use it for various purposes. Be it a free time or working hours, except a very few people, all depend on this machine to get their jobs done. This guide has everything you need to know about the computer work hazards and the preventive techniques you need to follow to make your stay in front of the computer, trouble free. The ebook is divided into different chapters to explain every aspect of this subject. As you read through the book I suggest you to compare each of the recommended position or method with your current style of working or handling. This way you can make sure that you are in the right path.

I have come across some common worries shared by people who have to sit for long hours in front of the computer.

- Is there a term called overuse of computers? If so, where do I draw the line?
- If I have to use it on a daily basis, how many hours of my presence in front of this machine is recommended?
- Will I be able to finish my work if I am to follow my recommended time schedule?

You can find answer to lot of such questions while reading through this book.

Chapter 1

Positioning Your Body

Before discussing on how to set your computer workstation, let's have a look at the concept of neutral body positioning. This can be defined as a comfortable working posture with a natural alignment of all your joints from head to toes. This method of neutral positioning helps you reduce the stress and strain on the muscles, tendons, and skeletal system thus reducing the risks of developing a musculoskeletal disorder (MSD). If you are a person who would like to maintain neutral body postures while working at the computer workstation, then you should be considering the following instructions:

- Ensure that your hands, wrists, and forearms are in a row, straight, and almost parallel to the floor.
- Ensure that your head and torso are in-line with head slightly bent forward, facing towards the front, and balanced.
- Ensure that your shoulders are at ease with upper arms hanging normally at the sides of your body.
- Ensure that your elbows are close to your body and bent between 90 and 110 degrees. Fig. 1 - Elbow angle

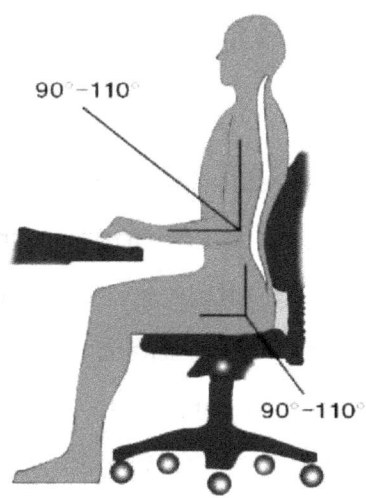

o The feet should be either supported by a footrest or should be relaxing on the floor.

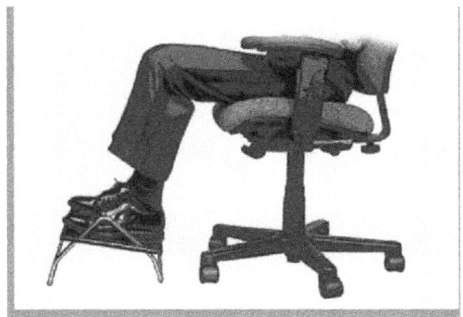

Fig. 2 - Footrest

o While leaning back or sitting in a vertical position, ensure that your back is supported fully with firm hold on the lumbosacral area.

o Your seat should be well padded in order to support your hips and thighs.

o Ensure that your knees and hips are in almost the same height with your feet slightly forward.

Even though you are positioned in the best of the postures at your workstation, it is not healthy to continue in that posture for long hours. It is ideal to change your position every now and then. The following are some tips to reduce your strain from continuing in the same posture in front of your computer.

- o Your chair and backrest have to be adjusted at regular intervals.
- o Your fingers, hands, arms, and torso need to be stretched periodically.

You need to stand up, stretch your back muscles, and stroll around for a few minutes now and again. Fig.3 – workspace dimensions

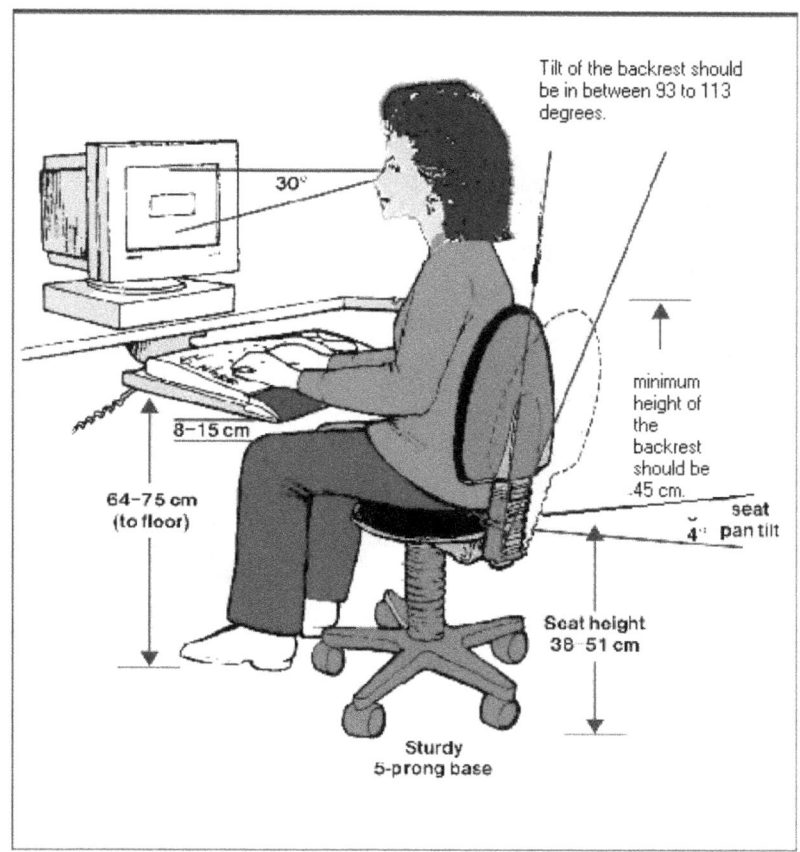

Let's now see some examples of changes in body postures that ensure neutral body positioning.

Vertical Sitting Posture

The neck and torso of the user are more or less vertical and in a row, the thighs are almost horizontal, with vertically positioned lower legs.

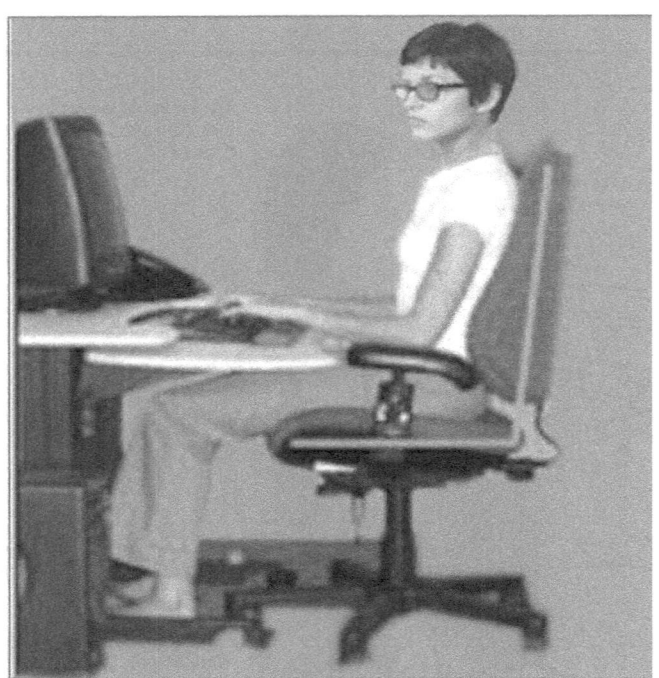

Fig.4 - Vertical Sitting Posture

Traction Posture

The legs, torso, neck, and head of the user are more or less in a row and vertical. The body weight of the user is either shared by both the legs or may elevate to a single leg.

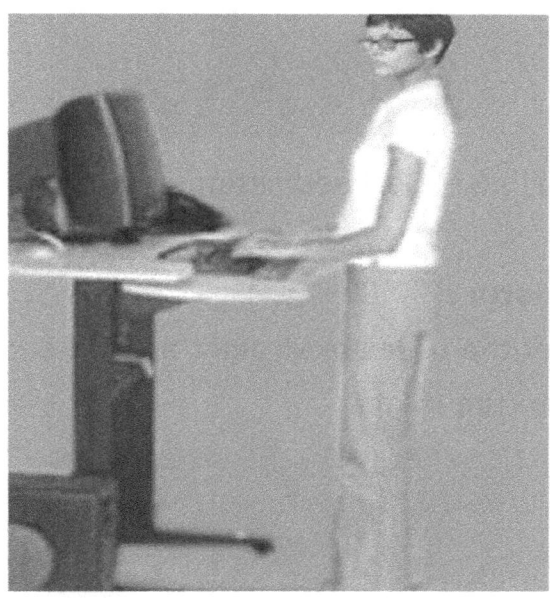

Fig. 5 – Traction posture

Declined Sitting Posture

The thighs of the user are inclined, the buttocks are higher than the knee and the angle between the thighs and the torso is greater than 90 degrees. The torso is vertical or slightly stretched out and the legs are vertical.

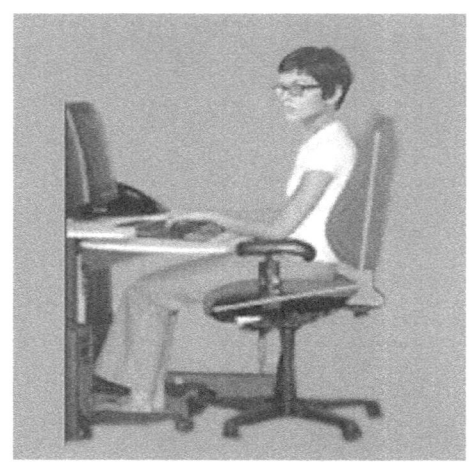

Fig.6 – Declined sitting posture

Reclined Sitting Posture

The torso and neck of the user are straight and tilt back between 105 and 120 degrees from the thighs.

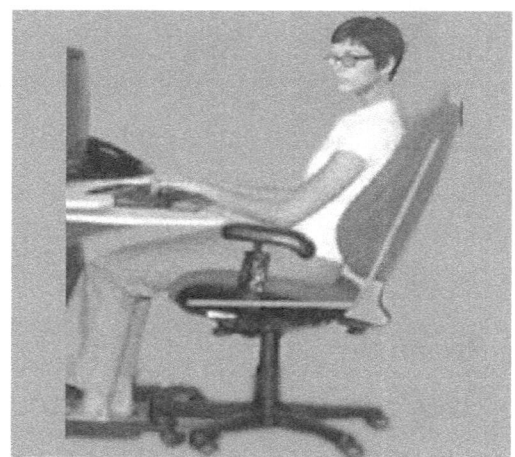

Fig.7 – Reclined sitting posture

Selection and Arrangement of the Components for the Workstation

The setting of the workstation, the selection and arrangement of the chair and other accessories, and his comfort in handling all the accessories of the desktop computer are the most vital factors that help the user to maintain a neutral body position. You need to check the following before starting to work on the system.

- o Check whether the workstation is set up well. The keyboard, the monitor, and your posture should be on a straight line so as to avoid any positional discomforts.
- o Never look up at the screen. Always adjust your chair as to look down at the screen.
- o The desktop should be at a convenient height with enough space for your computer and papers, if any.
- o The chair should give good support to your back with height-adjusting options.
- o The keyboard and the mouse mat should have a good wrist-rest.
- o For those who are copy typing, have a document holder so that you don't strain your neck and head too much.

Let us discuss how to select and arrange particular components for the workstation to help you carry out your work more professionally, contentedly and safely. The following sections explain how to select and arrange specific workstation components.

Monitors

Keyboards

Pointer/Mouse

Wrist/Palm Supports

Document Holders

Desks

Chairs

Telephones

Chapter 2

Monitors

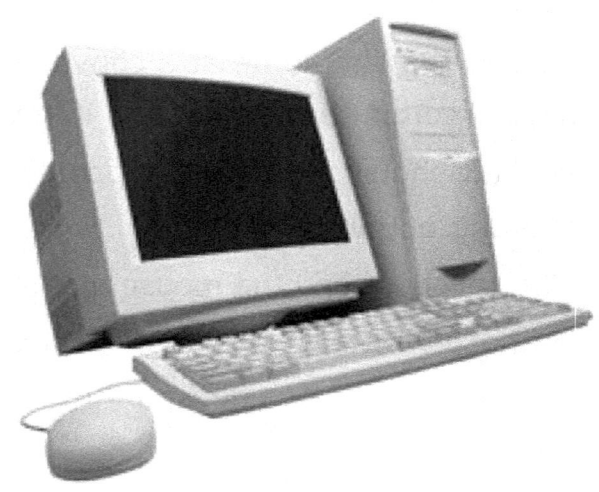

Fig. 7 – Desktop computer

Most of your time is spent looking at the monitor. Hence, utmost care should be given in choosing and appropriately placing it in your workstation. Suitable positioning of the monitor would help you reduce exposure to compelling exertions, inept postures, and overhead glare. Possible health issues like extreme exhaustion, eyestrain and related disorders like itching, sty, and power

variations of the eye lens, and neck and back pain can be avoided on proper selection of the monitor. The positioning of the monitor should be in concurrence with the other components like the keyboard, desk, and chair.

While using the monitor, ensure the following:

- Ensure that the monitor is in front of you and at least 20 inches away.
- Ensure that the top line of the screen is at or below your eye level.
- Ensure that the monitor is placed perpendicular to the window.

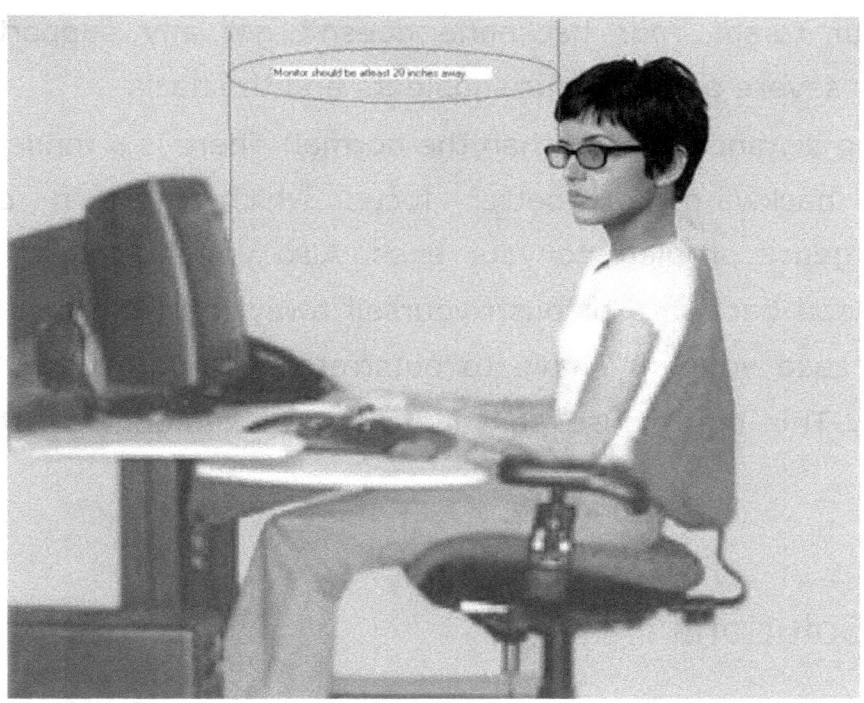

Fig 8 - The viewing distance

The viewing distance, viewing time, viewing angle, and viewing clarity have to be adjusted to get the best results without affecting your health.

Viewing Distance

Probable Risks

o You tend to lean forward or move backward thus positioning yourself awkwardly to have a better view of the monitor. Ensure that the monitors are neither too close nor too far so as to strain your eyes.

o Viewing distance longer than the normal: When you lean forward to view the monitor better, you are straining your eyes as well as your torso. Your backbone doesn't get any support that causes severe pain on your shoulders and the back.

o Viewing distance shorter than the normal: There is a tendency to move backward for better focus which in turn causes convergence problem to your eyes. Also you may tend to tilt your head backward or push yourself away from the monitor in which case you may have to outstretch your arms to do the typing. This may cause pain in your arms, fingers, wrist, and elbow.

Feasible Solutions

o Position yourself at a secure distance from the monitor wherein you can read all text without straining your eyes. Ensure that your head and torso are straight and your chair is firmly supporting the back. Ophthalmologists usually recommend a safe viewing distance between 20 and 40 inches (50 and 100 cm) from the eye to the front surface of the computer screen. If you still feel difficulty reading the text, do increase its font size.

- There should be ample desk space between the user and the monitor (table depth). If the desk space is not enough, here are some tips:

    1) Pull the desk away from the wall or the divider thus giving more space for the back of the monitor.
    2) Normally flat-panel displays are used which requires less desk space and are not as deep as the conventional monitor.

3) In order to make a deeper working surface, you can try installing an adjustable keyboard tray.

- Always remember to adjust the viewing distance between 20 and 40 inches.
- Flat-panel displays do not consume as much space as the conventional monitors

Viewing Angle–Height and Side-to-Side

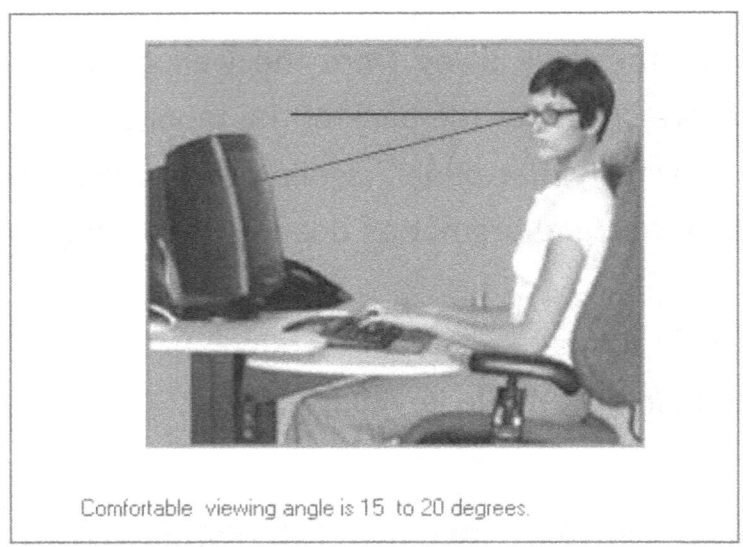

Comfortable viewing angle is 15 to 20 degrees.

Fig. 9 – viewing angle

Probable Risks

When you work in front of your computer for long hours with your head and neck turned to one side, you are sure to increase fatigue and pain in your neck muscles.

Feasible Solutions

- o While working on your computer, your head, neck, and torso should face forward and hence you need to be careful about positioning of the monitor. The ideal position is to place it directly in front of you. But, if that is not possible every time, the maximum tilt recommended is 35 degrees to the left or right.

o If your work is chiefly involved with printed matter, it will be ideal to place the monitor a little to the side with the printed matter just in front of you. The distance between the monitor and the printed matter should be minimal.

Probable Risks

Monitors that are placed too high or too low are not recommended for people who have to use computers for long hours per day. It affects the head, neck, shoulders, and the back, as they have to adjust their positions for better view of the monitor. In the long run, the muscles that support the head are fatigued due to these awkward postures.

Feasible Solutions

o Ensure that the top part of the monitor is either at the same level of your eyes or slightly below it. Also, the center of the monitor should be located 15 to 20 degrees below horizontal eye level.

o The entire visual area of the display screen should be located so that the downward viewing angle is never greater than 60 degrees when you are in any of the four reference postures. While in the reclining posture, the straightforward line of sight will not be parallel with the floor. This would increase the downward viewing angle. Also, very large monitors increase the angle.

o Do not to place the monitor above the other equipments like CPU or surge protector. The monitor would be too higher than your eyes that may increase the strain of your eyes, neck, and back.

- o The chair can be raised to lift your line of sight. Ensure that your feet get good support and your thighs can move freely under the desk.

Probable Risks

Those who use bifocal lenses normally view the monitor through the bottom portion of their lenses. In such case, they automatically tilt their head backward to have a better view of the monitor. And if the monitor is placed too high, the muscles that support their head easily get fatigued.

Feasible Solutions

The monitor can be lowered to avoid any kind of strain to the neck and eyes. The screen can be tilted a little upward for convenience.

Bifocal Lenses Cause Stress

- o The user is supposed to raise the height of the chair until the monitor can be viewed without having to tilt the head backwards. A footrest can be used and the keyboard can be raised a little for convenience.
- o Good single-vision lenses are available in the market with focal lengths designed for working in the computer. Viewing the monitor through the bottom portion of the lens can be avoided by using a pair of this single-vision lens.

Viewing Time

Probable Risks

If you view the monitor continuously for long hours without taking breaks, your eyes become dry and exhausted easily. You tend to blink less while working for long hours.

Feasible Solutions

- o Give rest to your eyes every so often by focusing on objects that are at a considerable distance from your seat like a painting on the wall around 20 feet away.
- o Periodically wet your eyes by blinking and looking at distant objects.
- o You tend to slow down in your work if you keep working for long hours on the computer. The ideal solution would be to take breaks in between and attend to other non-computer works like filing, making calls, or interacting with your customers. This gives good rest to your eyes.

Viewing Clarity

Probable Risks

Do not tilt monitors considerably either toward or away from the operator, as the objects on the screen may appear distorted making them illegible. And if the monitor is tilted back, there are chances of the overhead lights creating glare on the monitor. You tend to sit in different unhealthy positions to get a better view of the screen hence straining your eyes and the back.

Feasible Solutions

- o You can tilt the monitor somewhere between 10 to 20 degrees so that it is perpendicular to your line of sight. For this purpose, it is better to have a riser/swivel stand. If this is not possible, you can tilt the monitor back slightly by placing a book under the front edge. But to avoid glare in this case, do use a glare screen.
- o Monitor support surfaces should be user friendly by allowing the user to modify viewing distances and tilt and rotation angles.

Probable Risks

If the image that you view on the screen is of poor quality, your eyes have to strain more to view it properly. The distorted images may be due to electromagnetic fields caused by other electrical equipment located near computer workstations or due to dust accumulation. This is often accelerated by magnetic fields associated with computer monitors and can reduce contrast and degrade viewing conditions.

Feasible Solutions

- o Those equipments with electrostatic potentials more than +/- 500 volts should be kept away from your workstation.
- o Ensure that the monitor is dust free while in use.

Monitor Recipe

1. Always ensure that the screen is large enough for sufficient visibility. It is acceptable to use a 15 to 20-inch monitor. If the unit is very small, you will find it difficult to read the characters. If the unit is very large, you may require too much space.

2. Always ensure that the angle and tilt of the monitor can be adjusted without much effort.

3. For workstations with limited space, flat panel displays are preferred as they take less room on the desk.

Chapter 3

Keyboards

The selection and arrangement of the keyboard plays an important role in decreasing the exposure to awkward postures, repetition, and stress. While designing your computer workstation, you should keep in mind certain vital factors like the height of the keyboard, its distance, and the use. The placement of the keyboard should be

You should choose a keyboard and find a proper place matching with the other components like the pointer/mouse and wrist/palm rests.

Keyboard Guidelines

1) Ensure that the keyboard is placed directly in front of you.
2) Ensure that the elbows are close to your body and the shoulders are in relaxed position.
3) Ensure that your wrists are straight and in -line with your forearms.

Keyboard Placement – Height

Probable Risks

You tend to keep your shoulders, arm, and wrist in awkward positions if the keyboards, pointing devices, or working surfaces are placed too high or too. Normally, your wrists bent up when the keyboards are placed too low and you raise your shoulders to elevate your arms when the keyboards are placed too high. Such kind of awkward postures may lead to discomfort of the wrist, hand, and your shoulder.

Feasible Solutions

- o To maintain a neutral body posture, the height of the chair and the work surface need to be adjusted. Your elbows need to hang comfortably to the side of the body with the height almost same as the keyboard. The shoulders need to be in relaxed position and ensure that your wrists do not bend up or down or to either side while you are using the keyboard.
- o Ensure that the thickness of your work surface is not more than 2 inches.
- o Good keyboard trays with adjustable height and tilt giving enough space for leg and foot along with adequate space for other input devices like keyboard and pointer/mouse are available in the market if you find it difficult to adjust your work surface or your chair. While selecting a keyboard tray, ensure that it has all the mentioned features
- o The vertical position of the keyboard should be maintained within the recommended range. Its tilt can be raised or lowered using the keyboard feet to maintain straight, neutral wrist postures while making slight changes in arm angles.

Keyboard Placement – Distance

Probable Risks

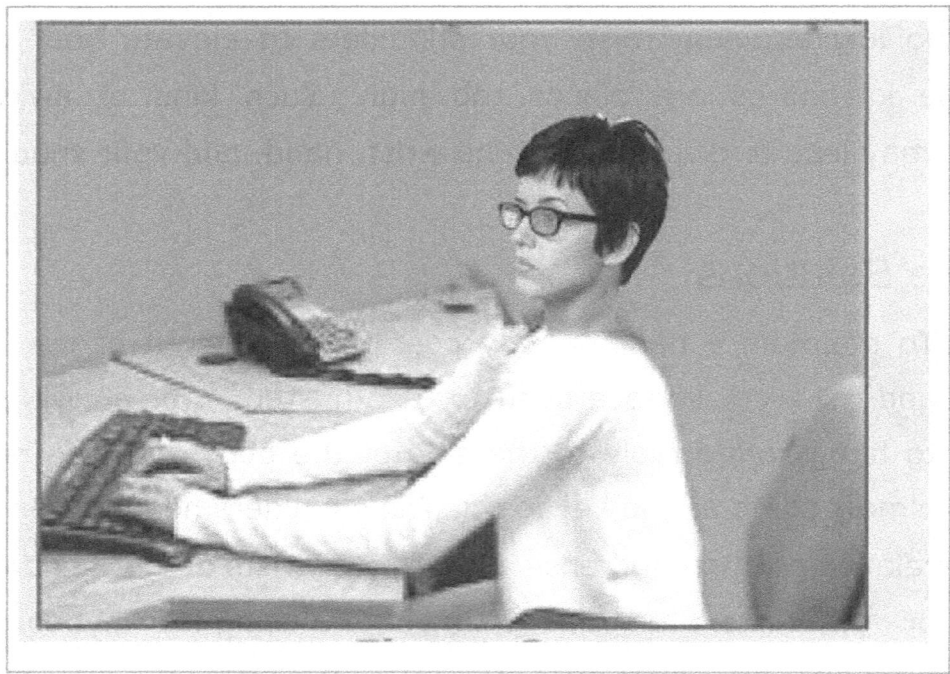

WRONG- Keyboard placed at an uncomfortable distance

Fig. 10

A keyboard user is forced to assume awkward postures such as reaching with the arms, leaning forward with the torso, and extreme elbow angles if the keyboard or pointer/mouse is placed too close or too far away from him. Studies have shown that such awkward postures generally lead to musculoskeletal disorders of the elbows, shoulders, hands, and wrists.

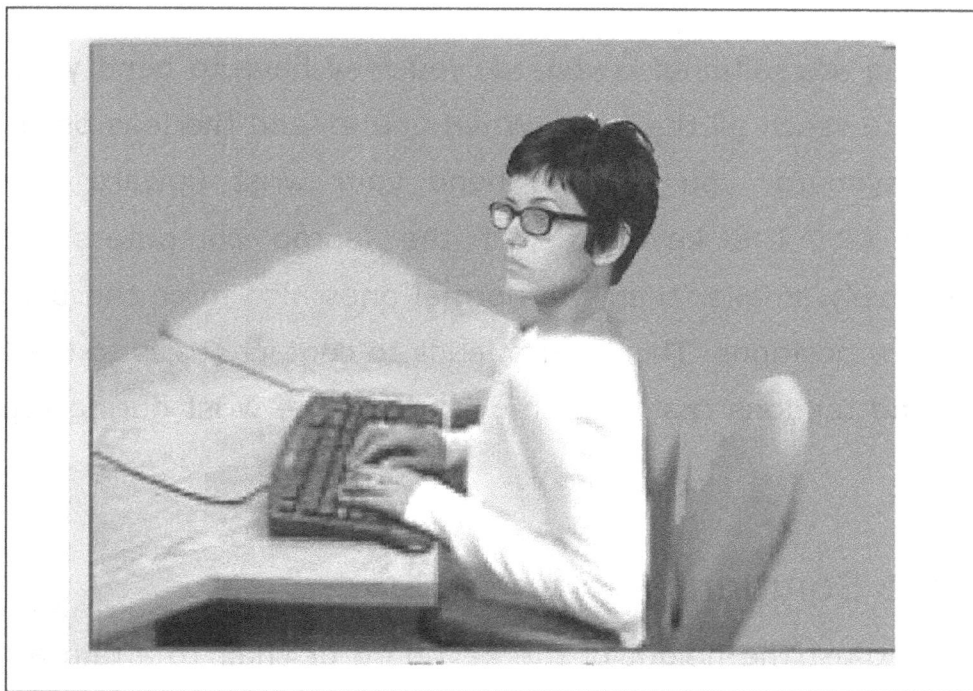

WRONG: Keyboard is too close

Fig. 11

Feasible Solutions

- o Ensure that the keyboard is placed directly in front of you at a distance that keeps your elbows close to your body with the forearms approximately parallel with the floor.
- o If the armrest of your chair doesn't allow sitting in a comfortable position or if your desk space is small, you can use a keyboard tray.

Design and Use

Probable Risks

While using a traditional keyboard, you may have to bend your wrists sideways to reach all the keys. When you extend the legs on the back of the keyboard, you tend to bend your wrist upward causing a keyboard tilt. The keyboards of the laptop computers that are comparatively smaller than the normal ones also force the user to sit in awkward positions. This in turn leads to contact stress to the tendon sheath and tendons that must move within the wrist during repetitive keying.

Feasible Solutions

- Adjust the height of the keyboard or chair to attain a neutral wrist posture thus reducing the awkward wrist angles.
- The user may even elevate the back or front of keyboards to achieve a neutral wrist posture. Normally, if the user is sitting in a position lower than that of the keyboard, a slight elevation made to the back of the keyboard would help maintain a neutral wrist. Similarly, if the user is typing with the keyboard in a lower position, raising the front of the keyboard may help maintain neutral wrist postures. If the keyboard feet tend to increase the bending of the wrist, do not use it.

- You can sit with neutral wrist postures by taking into account alternative keyboards. These can be provided on a case-by-case basis. It takes time to get used to such mechanisms. Though alternative keyboards help the users to maintain neutral wrist postures, studies have not yet provided enough information regarding its capability to avoid discomfort and injury.

o The size of the keyboard and spacing of the keys should be of appropriate size to suit majority of the customers. The recommended spacing between the centers of two keys horizontally is 0.71-0.75 inches (18-19 mm) and vertically is 0.71-0.82 inches (18-21 mm).

Keyboard Recipe

1. You can maintain neutral wrist postures by using split keyboard designs.

2. Keyboards with more adjustability options are often better than the others to maintain neutral wrist postures. There are keyboards with adjustable feet that can accommodate a wider range of keyboard positions and angles. Keyboards with adjustable feet on the front as well as the back will further aid adjustments.

3. Ensure that the cord connecting the keyboard and the CPU has ample length to let the user place both these components in a variety of convenient positions in the workstation. The recommended cord length is around six feet.

4. Consider a keyboard without a 10-key keypad if the task does not require one. If the task does require one occasionally, a keyboard with a separate 10-key keypad may be appropriate. Keyboards without keypads allow the user to place the mouse closer to the keyboard.

5. If you prefer to work with the keyboard tray, ensure that the size and shape of the keyboard matches with that of the tray.

6. It is always better to buy separate wrist rests than going for keyboards with built-in wrist rest.

7. If you have to work for prolonged hours with keyboards, detach them from the display screen. Do not use laptop for long hours of typing jobs.

Keyboard Tray Recipe

1. The width and depth of the keyboard trays should be large enough to accommodate the keyboard and any secondary devices, such as a mouse.

2. The minimum vertical adjustment range (for a sitting position) should be 22 inches to 28 inches from the floor, if you are working in the sitting position using the keyboard tray.

3. Ensure that your keyboard tray has adjustment mechanisms that lock into position without having to turn knobs. These are frequently over tightened, which can lead to stripped threads, or they may be difficult for some users to loosen.

While you are actually typing your wrists should not rest on anything, and should not be bent up, down, or to the side. Your arms should move your hands around instead of resting your wrists and stretching to hit keys with the fingers. NOTE : palm rests give you a place to rest your hands only when pausing from typing, NOT while you are typing. When you stop typing for a while, rest your hands on your lap or at. the sides instead of leaving them on the keyboard

Chapter 4

Your Mouse or Pointer

The pointing device or the mouse is now available in the market in different sizes, shapes, and configurations.   Apart from the conventional mouse, other pointing devices include touch pads, trackballs, fingertip joysticks, and pucks.   While designing a safe workstation, you should give great importance to selection and positioning of pointer/mouse.   Do keep in mind the following factors while evaluating your workstation.

1) Pointer Placement

2) Pointer Size, Shape, and Settings

Pointer/Mouse Guidelines

1) Ensure that the pointer/mouse is close to the keyboard.

2) Ensure that you use alternate hands while handling the pointer/mouse.

3) Learn and use the keyboard short cuts to reduce extended use.

Pointer Placement

Probable Risks

If the pointer/mouse is not placed near the keyboard, there are chances that your body will be exposed to awkward postures, contact stress, or forceful hand exertions while operating the device. If you continue to work in such postures for long hours, your shoulders and arms will be stressed out. For convenience you might sit with awkward wrist and shoulder postures that might lead to musculoskeletal disorders in the long run.

Feasible Solutions

o Select a particular position for the pointer/mouse so that you can maintain a straight, neutral wrist posture. If required, you may make slight adjustments in your chair, desk, keyboard tray, etc.

o If the keyboard tray/surface that you use does not have enough space for both the keyboard and the mouse, you can try out the following suggestions:

i) You can use a mouse platform over the keyboard that helps you to use the mouse above the 10-key pad.

ii) You can set up a mouse tray next to the keyboard tray.

iii) You can se a keyboard that has a pointing device, such as a touch pad, incorporated into it so that the work gets done even without the help of the mouse.

iv) You can try using a keyboard without a ten-key pad, which leaves more room for the pointer/mouse.

v) You can install keyboard trays that are big enough to accommodate both the keyboard and mouse.

vi) You can try a mouse pad with a wrist/palm rest to promote neutral wrist posture.

vii) You can substitute keystrokes hence depending less on the mouse, such as Ctrl+S to save, Ctrl+P to print etc.

Pointer Size, Shape, and Settings

Probable Risks

If the size and shape of the pointers that you choose are unsuitable, it may force you to sit in awkward postures, thereby increasing stress and hence overexertion. Generally, pointing devices that are too big or too small make the fingers to apply more force and bend the wrist to awkward positions. Also, if you operate a device designed for the right hand with your left hand, it leads to posture disorders that can create contact stress to the soft tissue areas in the palm of the hand. Contact stress leads to irritation and inflammation.

Feasible Solutions

- o The pointing device has to be selected to the fit the hand of the user who will be using it mostly. Pointing devices to fit right and left hands as well as small and large hands are available in the market. It is ideal to select a pointing device that is designed for either hand because you can switch from one hand to the other while operating the device hence giving rest to one hand at a time. Before selection of the device, it is better to test it and ensure proper fit and feel.
- o The size of the device matters and hence while selecting you need to ensure that you have to apply only a minimum force to generate movement. Normally puck devices should be small in size for using with single hand with a width of 1.5 to 2.5 inches, length of 2.5 to 4.5 inches, and a height of 1 to 1.5 inches.
- o It is better to reduce your dependence on the pointing device by using short cut keys and other options available on the

keyboard like page down thereby reducing the strain on hands.

- o Try out other pointing devices like joystick, touch pad, or trackball that fits your hand better and doesn't require bending the wrists when you grip the device. Remember to try out new products prior to selection and long-term use.

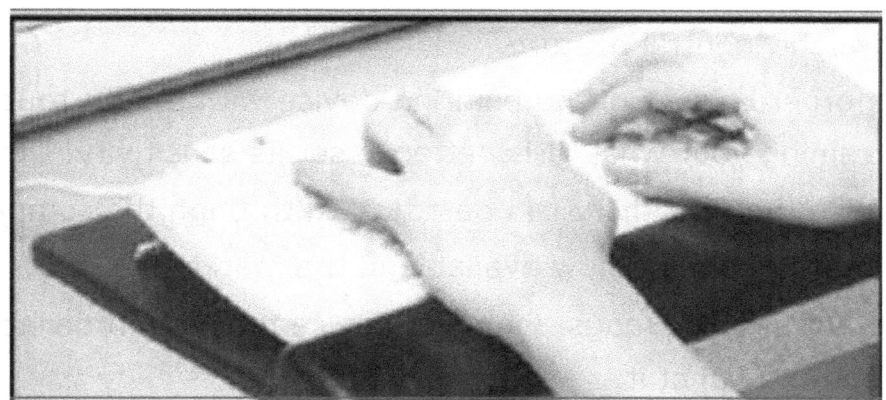

Fig. 11 –

Wrist / palm rest makes the positioning of the hand over the keyboard comfortable.

Probable Risks

If the sensitivity of the input device is not set properly, you tend to use more force and awkward hand postures to control it. For example, a very sensitive mouse may require excessive and extended finger force for good control. If the sensitivity of the mouse is not enough, you need to deviate the wrist in a wider angle to move the pointer to your desired place. When you exert your wrist forcefully for a long time or bend it repeatedly to place the pointer, your hand and arm muscles get fatigued increasing the risk of musculoskeletal injuries.

Feasible Solutions

- The speed of the pointer may be defined as the pace in which it moves on the screen when you move the pointing device with the hand. The pointing device that you select should be sensitive and fast enough so that you can comfortably adjust and control it as required. Also, the pointer should cover the entire screen of the monitor while your wrist is relaxed in a straight, neutral posture.
- In order to control the pointing device with a light touch without straining your wrist, it is better to set its sensitivity. Devices in which the sensitivity can be adjusted through the computer control panel are now available in the market.
- Do not grip the mouse/pointing device tightly in order to get good control of it.
- If you are using a trackball, ensure that its exposed surface are is not less that 100 degrees. It has to comfortably rotate in all directions for the user to try any combination of movement as required.

Mouse/Pointing Device Recipe

1. The mouse/pointing device should be selected based on the requirements of your job and your physical restrictions. Other than preference, there is no much difference between a mouse, trackball, and other pointing devices.

2. The cord of the mouse should be long enough to be conveniently placed near the keyboard. The shape and size of the mouse should be good enough to snug into the curve of your hand.

3. Among the different pointing devices, if you prefer a trackball for your work, remember not to select the ones that need your thumb for rolling its ball. This can cause discomfort and possible injury to the area around your thumb.

4. If the user's hands are small, then select a mouse that is smaller than the normal ones. But if multiple users are using it, then a normal-sized one should be retained.

5. Always go for a mouse that has good sensitivity adjustments and that can be used by both hands conveniently.

Wrist/Palm Supports

If your keyboard and mouse are arranged properly and appropriately, then you can say that your workstation is a comfortable and productive one. This comfort is intensified if you use wrist or palm rests. If used properly, wrist/palm supports reduce muscle activity while working on the computer and facilitates neutral wrist angle.

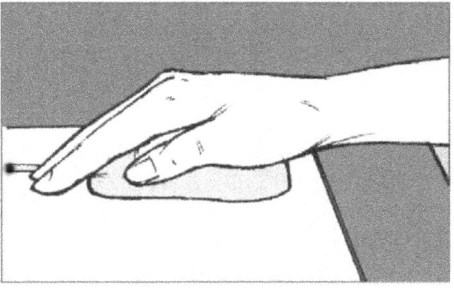

Fig. 12 - Palming the mouse makes the wrist straight.

Wrist Rest Guidelines

To keep the contact stress that can occur while typing and while using the mouse to a minimum, it is better to use a wrist rest so that you can maintain straight wrist postures.

Probable Risks

- The wrists tend to bend in a wider angle if you use the keyboard for long hours without using a wrist rest. As the angle of bend increases, the contact stress and irritation on tendons and tendon sheaths also increases. Professionals who depend more on keyboards to get their job done have to be very careful. The contact stress between the wrist of the user and the hard/sharp components in the workstation also increases.
- The motion of the wrist is slowed down while you are resting the wrist/palm on a support during the typing jobs that will in turn lead to awkward wrist postures.

Feasible Solutions

- Ensure that your hands are moving freely and are raised above the wrist/palm rest while using the keyboard. Also remember that the pad should be in touch with the palm of your hand and not your wrist while resting on the wrist rest.
- Ensure that these are part of a well-designed workstation.
- Do not frequently bend your wrists by adjusting other workstation components like that chair, desk, or the keyboard. See to it that your wrists are in a straight, neutral posture.
- The wrist support should be matched with the width, height, and slope of the front edge of the keyboard.

- The wrist/palm supports should be fairly soft and rounded to minimize pressure on the wrist. Ideally it should be at least 1.5 inches (3.8 cm) deep.

Wrist Rest Recipe

1. The shape, width, slope, and height of the wrist rest should match the front edge of the keyboard.

2. It would be better to use gel type materials for the padding that makes it soft and firm.

3. The recommended depth of the wrist rest is at least 1.5 inches (depth away from the keyboard). This helps to minimize contact pressure on the wrists and forearm.

Chapter 5

Document Holders   and Desk

While working with printed materials, document holders keep them near the user and the monitor. These can be positioned according to the convenience of the user depending on the type of the document and the task performed. Risk factors like awkward postures of the head and neck, fatigue, headaches, and eyestrain can be reduced by proper placement of these holders. If the monitor and keyboard are well placed and the user's chair is properly adjusted, then the holder can be placed without causing strain to the different body parts.

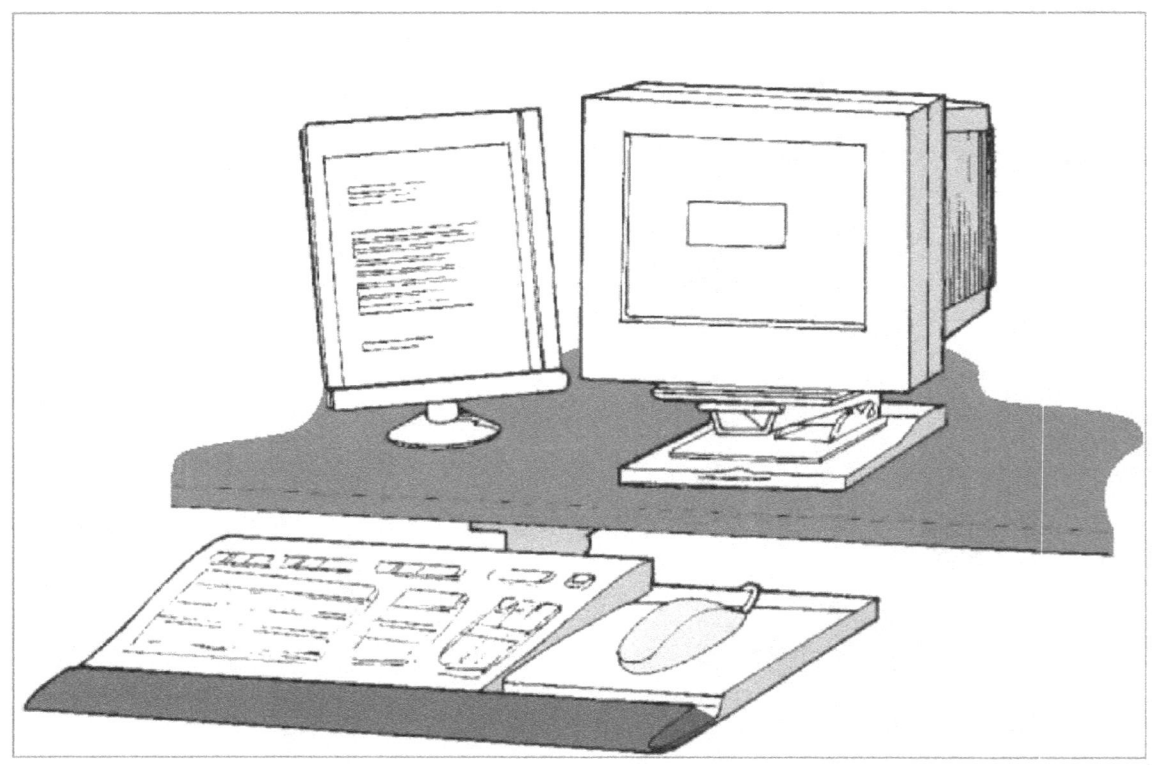

Fig. 3 - If your working mode necessitates looking to the document and the monitor very often, then place the document holder close to the computer as shown in the figure.

Document Holder Guidelines

The height and distance at which the printed materials are placed should be the same as that of the monitor.

Probable Risks

You tend to move your head and neck frequently or keep your head in awkward postures if the printed material that you are working is kept too far from the monitor. Such postures can lead to muscle fatigue and tenderness of the head, neck, and shoulders.

Feasible Solutions

o Ensure that the document holders that you use can place the documents at almost the same height and distance as the monitor. Even if you have to work on a big textbook, ensure that the holder is stable enough for that purpose.

o In fact, you get good document holders in the market that can be placed directly below the monitor. This gives a powerful writing surface if at all written entries are required, and hence decreases the frequent motion of your head, neck and back.

o Ensure that task lighting on the document does not create glare on the monitor.

Document Holder Recipe

1. It is better to go for document holders that are stable so that it stays firmly throughout your work. The height, position, distance, and viewing angle of the document holder should be easily adjustable by multiple users.

2. If your job involvement is more with the monitor, then prefer a document holder that can sit next to the monitor at its same height and distance.

3. A holder that can be placed conveniently between the monitor and the keyboard should be preferred if your job involves accessing the document frequently (such as writing on the document).

Desks

Before selecting a desk for your computer workstation, you should keep in mind its design and space. It should provide enough leg space, adequate space for other components and accessories and should help you minimize awkward postures and exertions. The installation, setup, and configuration of relaxed and productive workstations involves the following considerations:

- o   Desk or work surface areas
- o   Areas under the desk or work surface

Desk Quick Tips

- Ensure that the desk surface is capable of keeping the monitor directly in front of at a distance of at least 20 inches away.
- Do not keep items like CPU under the desk.
- The desk should allow you to work in various comfortable postures.

Desk or Work Surface Areas

Probable Risks

When the desk doesn't have enough space to accommodate all the components and accessories, you tend to place them in unfavorable positions. This in turn leads to awkward postures when you have to access a pointer/mouse or look at a monitor that is placed to the side.

Feasible Solutions

- Ensure that at least your mouse and keyboard are placed conveniently so that you don't have to sit in awkward positions every time you access them.
- Ensure that your work surface allows you to see the screen at a distance of at least 20 inches (50 cm), and position it to achieve the appropriate viewing angle, which is generally directly in front of you.
- Frequently used devices such as keyboard, phone, and mouse should be kept in the most easily accessible positions.

Probable Risks

There are some workstations where the desks and certain equipments have hard edges that usually touch the arm or wrist of the user. This, in the long run, may lead to contact stress affecting the nerves and blood vessels, causing tingling and sore fingers.

Feasible Solutions

Reasonably priced materials like pipe insulation can be padded on the hard edges of the table to reduce contact stress. Also use wrist rest and select only furniture with rounded desktop edges.

Probable Risks

Discomfort and inefficient performance of the computer operator may be due to insufficient clearance under the work surface. Some common discomforts are Shoulder, back, and neck pain due to the long distance of the users from computer components, causing them to reach to perform computer tasks; and generalized fatigue, circulation restrictions, and contact stress due to limitation of movement and inability to frequently change postures.

Feasible Solutions

- o Give enough clearance space for users to frequently change working postures. Items like files, CPUs, books, and storage should not be kept there.
- o Ensure that the clearance spaces under all working surfaces accommodate at least two of the three seated reference working postures, one of which must be the upright-seated posture.

Probable Risks

Too high or too low desk surfaces can lead to awkward postures such as extending your arms to reach the keyboard or raising your shoulders to get the job done. This may lead to muscular fatigue of the arms and shoulders.

Feasible Solutions

- o Risers like boards or concrete blocks can be inserted under the desk legs to lift the work surface.
- o Certain conventional desks have center drawers that block your thigh space. This can be removed for free movement of your thighs.
- o Cutting off the legs of the desk, if required can lower the work surfaces. If this does not work, the chair can be rose a little depending on the height of the user. A footrest, if necessary, can be used to support the user's feet.
- o Always select height-adjustable desks. Normally, the desk should be between 20-28 inches (50-72 cm) high.

Desk and Work Surface Recipe

1. Ensure that the desk area is deep enough to accommodate a monitor placed at least 20 inches away from your eyes.

2. It is recommended that the desk should have a work surface large enough to accommodate a monitor and a keyboard. Normally, a desk with a depth of about 30 inches is used to accommodate these items.

3. The height of the desk should be adjustable between 20 inches and 28 inches while the user is in sitting position. The desk surface should

be at about the height of your elbow while sitting with your feet flat on the floor. Adjustability between seated and standing heights is desirable.

4. Ensure that the user has sufficient space to place the frequently used items like keyboard, mouse, and monitor directly in front of you.

5. Your desk should provide enough space underneath for your legs while sitting in all convenient positions. The minimum under-desk clearance depth should be 15 inches for your knees and 24 inches for your feet. There should be at least 20 inches clearance width.

6. When you purchase a desk with a fixed height, ensure that you have a keyboard tray to provide enough height adjustment to suit multiple users.

7. Avoid glass tops and glossy desktops. Ensure that your desktops have a matte finish to minimize glare.

8. At areas where your arms touch the work surfaces, ensure that there are no sharp edges. Rounded or sloping surfaces are preferable.

9. The leading edge of the work surface should be wide enough to accommodate the arms of your chair, usually about 24 inches to 27 inches. If the space is lesser than this, it will interfere with armrests and restrict your movement. This is to be kept in mind especially while working in four-corner work units.

Work Space

The clearance space under the work surface should have adequate legroom for the user while positioned in the upright-seated posture and at least one of the other seated reference postures. Methods 1 or 2 can be applied to achieve this.

Method 1 - Upright and Reclined Seated Postures

When in a seated posture where the top of the legs is about parallel with the floor, the dimensions that represent clearances that accommodate the majority of the users are as mentioned below. The majority of the users consist of 5th percentile female to 95th percentile male.

Minimum dimensions

- o 20 inches (52 cm) wide.
- o 17 inches (44 cm) deep at knee level.
- o 24 inches (60 cm) deep at foot level.
- o 4 inches (10 cm) high at the foot.

Variable dimensions ("rollover" the image)

Height is adjustable between 20 and 27 inches (50 and 69 cm) near the user.

Method 2 - Upright, Reclined, and Declined Seated Postures

The following dimensions accommodate the largest operator clearance spaces (5th percentile female to 95th percentile male). Thus, specifications conforming to Method 2 will meet Method 1 requirements. This method also includes postures where the knee is slightly lower than the buttocks (declined-seated).

Minimum dimensions

See above

Variable dimensions ("rollover" the images)
- o Adjustable between 20 and 28 inches (50 and 72 cm) high at the hip.
- o Adjustable between 20 and 25 inches (50 and 64 cm) high near the user's knee.

Chapter 6

Chairs

While talking about a safe and productive computer workstation, the topic of a well-designed and appropriated-adjusted chair comes to our mind naturally. Being an inevitable part of a good workstation, chair offers essential support to the back, legs, buttocks, and arms, along with reducing exposures to awkward postures, contact stress, and forceful exertions. The advantages of using a chair with increased adjustability include ensuring a better fit for the user, providing sufficient support in a variety of sitting postures, and allowing variety of convenient sitting positions throughout the workday. If more than one person is using the chair per day, these points have more relevance. Before selecting a particular chair, try out different ones and finalize on the one that gives the best support. To ensure that the chair will provide adequate support, it is important that you try out different chairs before purchasing one. To create a safe and dynamic workstation, the following parts of the chair have to be observed in detail before selection.

- o Backrest
- o Seat
- o Armrest
- o Base

The chair should be adjusted while placing the monitor, keyboard and desk in your workstation.

Chair Guidelines

- o Ensure that the backrest of your chair corresponds to the natural curvature of your spine providing enough support to the lumbar region.
- o Ensure that the seats of your chair are comfortable enough to allow your feet to rest flat on the floor or footrest.
- o Ensure that the armrests of your chair are soft allowing your shoulders to relax and elbows to stay close to your body.
- o Ensure that your chair has a five-leg base with rollers that allow it to move easily on the floor.

Backrest of the chair

Probable Risks

If the backrest of the chair is not designed properly with inadequate size, material, and positioning, the back support will not be sufficient. This would lead to inappropriate postures that cause back pain and fatigue. A chair without

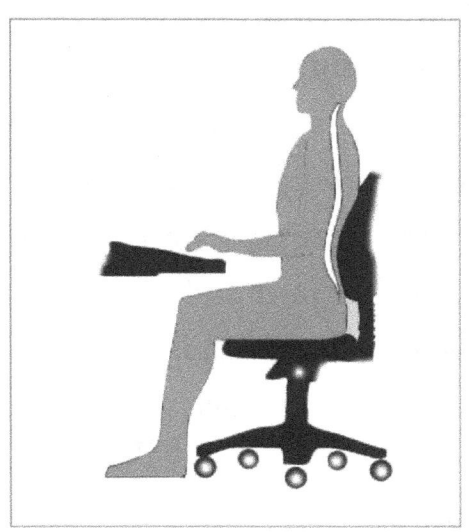

Fig. 14 – The backrest position

suitable or appropriate backrest will fail in supporting your lumbar spine and won't maintain the natural S-shape curvature of the spine.

Feasible Solutions

- o Roll up a towel at the lumbar region or place a removable back support cushion for a temporary support if the chair that you use currently doesn't provide a good lumbar support. This would help you maintain the natural curve of the spine.

- o You can try using a chair with easily adjustable backrest and which supports the back in all your convenient seating postures. A backrest should have the following features:

  - ☺ The backrest should have a good lumbar support with adjustable height options for fitting the lower back in different postures. Ensure that the outward curve of the backrest should fit into the small of the back.

  - ☺ The backrest should have an adjustment that allows the user to recline at least 15 degrees from the vertical. The backrest should lock in place or be tension adjustable so that adequate resistance is ensured to the lower back movement.

- ⏰ Shorter users can sit with their backs against the backrest without worrying about their knees touching the front edge of the seat pan with the help of a device that enables to move forward and backward. Taller users can sit with their backs against the backrest while supporting their thighs and buttocks fully.

Probable Risks

Too high chairs force the users to work with their feet unsupported and make them move forward in the chair to a position where the back gets zero support which makes it even more difficult for them to maintain the S-shape of the spine. If the user sits continuously in such postures, it can cause fatigue, restricted circulation, swelling, numbness, and pain.

Feasible Solutions

- o Do make use of a footrest that gives good support to the feet if your seat cannot be lowered.
- o The seat pan of your chair should be adjustable and of appropriate size to provide support to your body in all your convenient postures. See to it that the seat has the following features:
  - ⏰ The height of the seat should be adjustable especially when there are multiple users. It is ideal if the entire sole of the user's feet can be rested on the floor with the back portion of the knee slightly higher that the seat of the chair.

- The seat has padded and a rounded, "waterfall" edge.
- The width of the seat should accommodate almost all the hip sizes, at least the majority. For larger users, those with oversize seat pans should be provided.

Probable Risks

It is very uncomfortable for the user to sit in a seat pan that is inappropriately sized. It fails to give enough support to the legs and restrict the whole body movements of the user. Shorter ones place more pressure on the buttocks of the taller users and longer ones place more pressure on the knees of the shorter users minimizing the back support. One that is too small can restrict movement and provide inadequate support. Prolonged use can restrict blood flow to the legs and create irritation and pain.

Feasible Solutions

o The depth of the seat pan should be adjustable to support taller users adequately simultaneously allowing shorter users to sit with full support to their back. It should also provide support for most of the thigh without contact between the back of the user's knee and the front edge of the seat pan.

o Always use a footrest, which elevates the knee slightly to relieve pressure on the back of the leg.

o Use a chair that is sized to fit small or large users. This is very important if multiple users share the chair.

Probable Risks

Most users tend to sit in awkward postures and thus lack adequate support, if the armrests they use are not adjustable. Let's discuss the negative points of such armrests:

- o Armrests that are too low force you to lean over to the side to rest one forearm which in turn results in uneven and awkward postures, fatiguing the neck, shoulders, and back.

- o Armrests that are too high force you to sit with raised shoulders resulting in muscle tension and fatigue in the neck and shoulders.

- o Armrests that are too wide force you to reach with the elbow and bend forward for support. This results in pulling the arm from the body and leads to muscle fatigue in the shoulders and neck.

- o Armrests that are too close restrict movement in and out of the chair.

- o Armrests that are too large or inappropriately placed may interfere with the positioning of the chair. If the chair cannot be placed close enough to the keyboard, you may have to reach and lean forward in your chair. This in turn leads to fatigue and strain the lower back, arm, and shoulder.

- o Armrests that are made of hard materials or that have sharp corners can irritate the nerves and blood vessels located in the forearm. This will create pain or tingling in the fingers, hand, and arm.

Feasible Solutions

Some chairs come with armrests that give more discomfort that comfort while working on the computer. Some interfere with your workstation and some others cannot be adjusted properly. Try removing such armrests or at least stop using such armrests. While selecting chairs with armrests, check whether they can be adjusted according to your postures so that they give good support to your lower arm while allowing the upper arm to be close to the body. Armrests that can be properly adjusted should have the following features:

- o They should have ample width for the users to get in and get out of the chair easily.
- o They should be close enough to support your lower arms keeping your upper arms close to your torso.
- o They should be low enough keeping your shoulders relaxed while working on the computer.

- o They should be high enough to support your lower arms when positioned comfortably at your sides. If the armrests are too low and you find it difficult to adjust them, add padding to the top of the armrests.
- o They should be large enough to support most of your lower arm. Moreover, ensure that they are small so that they do not interfere with your chair positioning.
- o Ensure that the armrests are made of soft material and have blunt edges.

It is not necessary that all users should keep armrests to their chairs. It depends on the amount of hours the user spends on the system per day, whether the user has suffered from or is suffering from musculoskeletal disorder (MSD), or whether the user prefers to work with armrests on the chair. But, if you have already decided to have a pair for your chair, do consider all the above-mentioned points before selecting the product.

Probable Risks

- o If the number of legs of your chair are four or less than four, the support and balance it gives the user will be lesser and hence there are chances of the chair bending and hence the user falling down.

- o If the casters used for the chair are not good or if the chair doesn't have casters, the user might find it difficult to position the chair with respect to the desk. Inappropriate choice of casters, or a chair without casters, can make positioning the chair in relation to the desk difficult. This may result in the user bending to access the different components that in turn might lead to muscular strain and fatigue.

Feasible Solutions

- o Ensure that your chair has a strong, five-legged base.
- o The casters of the chair should go with the flooring of the workstation. Do ensure that the casters of your chair are proper enough.

Chair Recipe

1. The chair that you select for your workstation should be easily adjustable.

2. Ensure that your chair has a strong base with five legs with casters that are good enough to roll over the floor or carpet.

3. The chair should revolve 360 degrees sot that the user can access items around the workstation without twisting and straining.

4. It is recommended that the height of the seat is at least 16 inches.

5. The length of the seat pan should be between 15 inches and 17 inches.

6. The width of the seat pan should be at least 18 inches. It should have ample room for the user's thighs.

7. The edges of the chair should be padded and shaped with soft, but firm material for good support.

8. It is recommended that the minimum adjustable tilt of the seat pan should be in the range of 5 degrees, both forward and backward.

9. Try to avoid extremely contoured seats because they restrict different convenient sitting postures and are uncomfortable for many users.

10. Ensure that the front edge of the seat pan is rounded in a 'waterfall' fashion.

11. Check whether the material used for the seat pan and back is firm, breathable, and resilient.

12. The depth of the seat pan should be adjustable. Do not go for chairs in which only the back can be tilted forward and backward because they don't provide adequate adjustment for multiple users. There are chairs with seat pans that can slide forward and backward and have a fixed back. There are some other chairs in which the position of the seat pan is fixed and the backrest moves horizontally

forward and backward, so that the effective depth of the seat pan can be adjusted.

13. The height and width of the backrest should be at least 15 inches and 12 inches respectively. It should be firm enough to provide lumbar support that matches the curve of your lower back.

14. The backrest of your chair should widen at its base and curve in from the sides to coincide with your body. Ensure that it does not meddle much with your arms.

15. The backrest should allow you to recline at least 15 degrees and should be able to lock into place for firm support.

16. The backrest should be high enough to support your upper trunk and neck/shoulder area. A headrest should be provided if the backrest reclines more than about 30 degrees from vertical.

17. The chair should have removable armrests and the distance between them should be adjustable. The distance between the armrests should be at least 16 inches.

18. The height of the armrests should be adjustable between 7 inches and 10.5 inches from the seat pan. It is better not to use fixed height armrests, especially for chairs with multiple users.

19. The length and width of the armrests should be large enough to support your forearm without meddling with the work surface.

20. The padding of the armrests should be firm and soft.

21. Normally, chairs for the workstation are designed for users weighing below 275 pounds. For users weighing above 275 pounds, the chair must be designed to support the extra weight.

I personally use the SteelCase Leap Chair Coach Edition, this chair retails for $2000.00, this should tell you how serious I am about working smarter.

My back aches ended the day I purchased this chair, I can not recommend it highly enough.

There are non Coach editions of the Leap Chair starting at $450

Another chair I would highly recommend is the Aeron by Herman Miller.

Chapter 7

Telephones

In today's competitive market, most of the jobs revolve around telephones and computers as key workstation components. Telephones are an inevitable part of the workstation because they add to the convenience of your work. Yet, this combination is very dangerous as you tend to use both the devices simultaneously which may lead to musculoskeletal disorders. The cords of the telephone can get tangled up hence causing the user to assume awkward postures.

Telephone Quick Tips

- If your job involves speaking over the phone for a long time, do use a speakerphone.
- Ensure that the speakerphone is close to you so that you don't have to reach it every time, which in turn causes strain.

Probable Risks in Placement and Use

If the telephone is placed too far away from the user, it causes strain on the shoulder, arm, and neck due to repeated reaching.

Feasible Solutions

- Let your telephone be placed in the primary or secondary work zone, depending on usage patterns. Thus you can avoid reaching it repeatedly, reducing the possibility of injury.
- Ensure that the cord of your telephone is out of the work area so that it does not create a tripping hazard.

Probable Risk

Some users do not want to waste their time when they have to use the phone while working on the computer. Hence they keep the phone pinched between their head and shoulder thus talking over the phone and working on the computer simultaneously. This may cause stress on the neck and especially the ears as they are pressed between the head and shoulders during the entire conversation.

Feasible Solution

If you have to spend a lot of time on the phone while using the computer, it is ideal to use a "hands-free" headset. If your co-workers do not have a problem, speakerphone is yet another appropriate solution provided the volume is adjusted for your audibility only.

Telephone Recipe

1. Always use a telephone with a "hands free" headset if your job at the workstation involves more of manual tasks such as typing so that you don't strain your neck and head while doing both the tasks simultaneously.

2. Use a telephone that has a "hands-free" feature.

3. Ensure that your "hands-free" headsets have volume control options.

Chapter 8

What We Have Learned

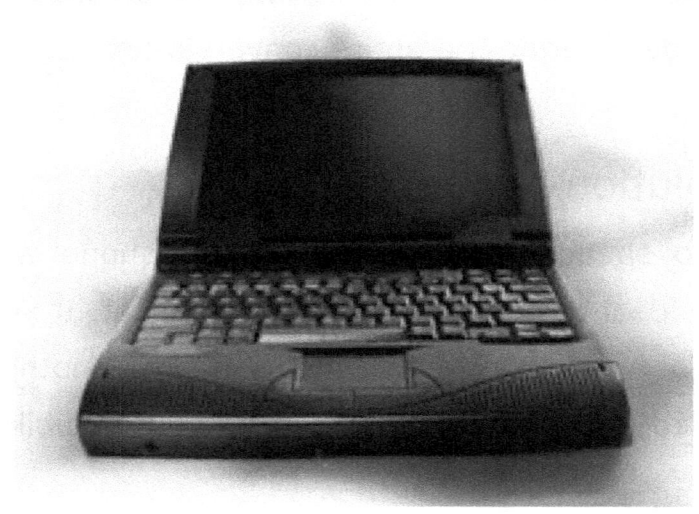

Fig. 15- A laptop is not recommended for long time usage.

Due to its special design, size, and shape, a laptop workstation creates special challenges. All the points discussed about the different components of the computer workstation are applicable to laptops too. Users possessing laptops can go through these points for additional information.

Questionnaire

We now present a checklist that will help you create a safe, sound, and relaxed workstation. You can try using it in combination with the purchasing guide checklist. There are two options – 'Yes' and 'No'. The questions relate to different topics like working postures, seating, keyboard, monitors, accessories, work area and some general questions. If the response is 'no', it means that a problem exists. You can refer to the above-mentioned information to get ideas about how to evaluate and manage the problem.

WORKING POSTURES

1. Do your head and neck need to be upright, or in-line with the your torso (not bent down/back)? If your answer is "no", then refer to the section on Monitors, Chairs and Work Surfaces.

2. Do the head, neck, and trunk need to be facing forward without twisting? If your answer is "no", then refer to the section on Monitors or Chairs.

3. Does your trunk have to be perpendicular to the floor (you may lean back into backrest but not forward)? If your answer is "no", then refer to the section on Chairs or Monitors.

4. Do your shoulders and upper arms need to be relaxed and in-line with the torso, normally about perpendicular to the floor (but not

elevated or stretched forward)? If your answer is "no", then refer to the section on Chairs.

5. Do the upper arms and elbows need to be close to the body and not extended outward? If your answer is "no", then refer to the section on Chairs, Work Surfaces, Keyboards, and Pointers.

6. Do your forearms, wrists, and hands need to be straight and in -line (forearm at about 90 degrees to the upper arm)? If your answer is "no", then refer to the section on Chairs, Keyboards, Pointers.

7. Do the wrists and hands need to be straight (not bent up/down or sideways toward the little finger)? If your answer is "no", then refer to the section on Keyboards, or Pointers.

8. Do both the thighs need to be parallel to the floor and the lower legs to be perpendicular to floor (thighs may be slightly elevated above knees)? If your answer is "no", then refer to the section on Chairs or Work Surfaces.

9. Can your feet rest flat on the floor or should they be supported by a stable footrest? If your answer is "no", then refer to the section on Chairs or Work Surfaces.

SEATING (Chair)

10. Does the backrest of the chair support your lower back?

11. Does the seat width and depth have the capacity for the specific user (seat pan not too big/small)?

12. Is the seat pan of your chair too long to press against the back of your knees and lower legs? If your answer is 'yes', review the section on Chairs.

13. Is your seat cushioned properly, rounded, and blunt with a "waterfall" front?

14. Do the armrests of your chair support both forearms while working on the computer without meddling with your movement?

If your answer is "no" for any of these questions other than question number 12, then refer to the section on Chairs.

KEYBOARD

15. Are the platforms for the keyboard/input device stable and large enough to hold a keyboard and an input device?

16. Are the input devices (mouse or trackball) located right next to your keyboard so that they can be accessed and used without having to reach them?

17. Can the input devices be easily activated with their size and shape fitting your hand (not too big/small)?

18. Does your workstation ensure that your wrists and hands do not rest on sharp or hard edges?

If your answer is "no", then refer to the section on Keyboards, Pointers, or Wrist Rests.

MONITOR

19. Is the top of the monitor screen at or below your eye level so that you can read it without bending your head or neck down/back?

20. Can the user with bifocals/trifocals read the screen without bending the head or neck backward?

21. Does the distance of the monitor allow you to read the screen without leaning your head, neck, or trunk forward/backward?

22. Is the monitor positioned directly in front of you so that you don't have to twist your head or neck?

23. Do you ensure that glare (for example, from windows, lights) is not reflected on your screen that makes you sit in awkward postures so as to view the screen better?

If your answer is "no", then review the section on Monitors or Lighting/Glare.

WORK AREA (Desk and Workstation)

24. Between the top of the thighs and your computer table, do you have enough room or your thighs (thighs are not trapped)?

25. Do you ensure that your legs and feet have sufficient clearance space under the work surface so that you can get close enough to the keyboard/input device?

ACCESSORIES

26. Is your document holder stable and large enough to hold documents?

27. Is your document holder placed at about the same height and distance as the monitor screen so that there is little head movement, or need to re-focus, when you look from the document to the screen?

28. Is your wrist/palm rest padded and free of sharp or square edges that push on your wrists?

29. Does your wrist/palm rest allow you to keep your forearms, wrists, and hands straight and in-line when using the keyboard/input device?

30. While doing telephone and computer tasks simultaneously, do you keep your head upright (not bent) and your shoulders relaxed (not elevated)?

If your answer is "no" for question from 24 through 30, then review the section on Work Surfaces, Document Holders, Wrist Rests or Telephones.

GENERAL

31. Do your workstation and equipment have sufficient adjustability that ensures your safe working posture while allowing you to make occasional changes in posture when you work on your computer?

32. Are your computer workstation, components, and accessories maintained in serviceable condition and do they function properly?

33. Are your computer tasks planned in a way that allows you to vary tasks with other work activities, or to take micro-breaks, or recovery pauses while at the computer workstation?

If your answer is "no", then refer to the section on Chairs,
Work Surfaces, or Work Processes.

Chapter 9

Work Process and
Recognition

Untill now we have been discussing the different ways by which, you get affected by sitting in front of the computer for long hours and the different options that you can try to avoid them. Though you follow all those recommendations and solutions to the best of your capability, there are still other kinds of hazards like task organization that can strengthen the effect of other risk factors, such as repetition. Moreover, if you fail to recognize early warning signs, they may lead to small problems to develop into serious injuries. If you concentrate more on task organization factors and medical awareness, it can help you to minimize the risk of developing musculoskeletal disorders (MSDs) and stop further advancement to injury.

Let us discuss two important factors in this context.

(i) Prolonged Periods of Activity

(ii) Medical Awareness and Training

Prolonged Periods of Activity

Probable Risks

Computers are a part of life these days. They play the role of a teacher, mailman, newspaper, and television.

The software industry also provides jobs to many people. Computer work, when viewed from a total body outlook, may seem to be an effortless activity, whether it's for a job or for fun. But, if the user performs highly repetitive tasks for prolonged periods in the same posture, it may cause discomforts in localized areas of the body. For instance, everybody depends on the mouse while working on the computer. If this is used for a few minutes, it should not be a problem for most users. But performing this task continuously for more than a few uninterrupted hours can expose the small muscles and tendons of the hand to hundreds or even thousands of activations (repetitions). The user may not get enough time between activations for rest and recovery, which can cause localized fatigue, wear and tear, and injury. Similarly, if the user maintains static postures continuously, such as viewing the monitor without taking a break, it can fatigue the muscles of the neck and shoulder that support the head.

Feasible Solutions

1) Try to vary your tasks and workstations so that you get ample time to recover from the outcome of your activity. Different ways are being practiced to provide recovery time for overused muscles.

2) Design your workstation in such a way that you can easily change your working postures according to your convenience. It is always safe to select adjustable furniture for the workstation that allows you to shift to different seated postures every time you want to. This helps different muscle groups to provide support while others rest.

3) Your work area should be spacious enough to let you use the mouse with either hand alternately. Thus the tendons and muscles of the free hand get enough relaxation.

4) Reduce your dependence on the mouse and use more of shortcut keys. For example, you can use Ctrl+S to save, Ctrl+P to print etc. Certain jobs do require more dependence on the mouse. Users in such professions should learn to use more shortcut keys.

5) Jobs that involve more repeated tasks or prolonged static postures may lead to muscular strain. The users should forcefully take several short breaks or relaxed pauses. The users should stand, stretch, and move around during such breaks. This increases blood circulation and gives enough time for the muscles to relax.

6) Try to mix computer tasks and non-computer tasks alternately in all possible situations. This encourages the movement of different parts of the body by using different muscle groups.

Medical Awareness and Training

Probable Risks

Most of the users neither get a chance to go through a proper training to identify the risks and hazards nor do they realize effective work practices designed to reduce these hazards. Such people have more chances of getting affected because of their ignorance. Even though disorders like MSD affect them, they are not medically aware of the signs and symptoms and hence do not notice or address such issues. For instance, users who don't realize the hazards of awkward postures while working on the computer don't know how to take care of their pains and strains. Delay in realizing and diagnosing such discomforts may lead to severe injury.

Feasible Solutions

Everybody who uses computers is bound to acquire training on general ergonomic awareness based on the following issues:

- They should get trained on the aspects related to all the computer components exclusively, that generally increase discomfort or risk of injury
- They should be made aware of the different signs and symptoms of all kinds of discomforts caused by continuous computer usage so that they can identify these from the beginning and treat with appropriate medications.
- They should be given enough information on the methods of using and adjusting all the computer components correctly as well as the environmental factors.

Workstation Environment

You can have a better view of the monitor and see the images clearly if you take good care in selecting the right level of illumination and place it appropriately. Normally, brighter lighting or sources that cause glare on your monitor lead to eyestrain or headaches which may force you to work in awkward postures to have a better view of the screen. The comfort of the user and hence his productivity is related to the aeration and moisture levels in the workstation environment. We shall take a look at the 3 factors that affect the workstation environment.

- Lighting
- Glare
- Ventilation

Environment Quick Tips

1) You should design your office in such a way that the glare from overhead lights, desk lamps, and windows is reduced to a maximum.

2) Your office room should be designed in such a way as to maintain appropriate air circulation.

3) Do not sit directly under air conditioning vents that push air right on top of you.

Chapter 10

Lighting

Lighting is a very important aspect of a healthy working environment.
Do not take this section lightly, no pun intended!

1. The lighting at your workstation depends on the type of job you are involved in. Do use bright lights with a large lighted area while working with printed materials. Limit the brightness of light for computer tasks.

2. The user should be able to adjust the position and angle of the light sources, as well as their intensity levels.

3. To direct or diffuse the light, it should have a hood or filter.

4. The base of the light should be large enough to allow a variety of convenient positions or extensions.

Probable Risks

If the monitor is displayed with maximum brightness, you will have to strain your eyes more to view the objects on the screen clearly thus leading to eye fatigue.

Feasible Solutions

1) It is ideal to place lights parallel to your line of sight in different rows.

2) Try to use light diffusers so that you can do the desk jobs like writing, reading papers etc. while limiting direct brightness on the computer screen.

3) While using 4-bulb fluorescent light fixtures, it is ideal to remove the middle bulbs to reduce the brightness of the light to levels well suited with computer tasks, if diffusers or alternative light sources are not available.

Note: A standard florescent light fixture on a nine-foot ceiling with four, 40-watt bulbs will produce approximately 50 foot-candles of light at the desktop level.

4) You need to have good desk lighting for proper illumination while writing and reading tasks thus limiting brightness around monitors.

5) Generally, for paper tasks and offices with CRT displays, office lighting should range between 20 to 50 foot-candles. For LCD monitors, higher levels of light are usually needed for the same viewing tasks (up to 73 foot-candles).

Probable Risks

The light sources behind the display screen can create contrast problems, making it difficult to view the screen clearly.

Feasible Solutions

1) You can try using blinds or drapes on windows to eliminate bright light. The placement of blinds and furniture should be adjusted to allow light into the room, but not directly into your field of view.

Note: Vertical blinds are ideal for windows facing east/west directions and horizontal blinds are ideal for windows facing north/south directions.

2) Indirect or shielded lighting can be used wherever possible. Try to avoid intense or uneven lighting in your field of vision. You should also ensure that lamps have glare shields or shades to direct light away from your line of sight.

3) If the bright lights from open windows in your work area are at right angles with your computer screen, do change the orientation of your workstation.

Probable Risks

You may be affected with headaches and eye fatigue if the contrast between light and dark areas of the computer screen are high.

Feasible Solution

1) It is recommended to use well-distributed diffuse light for your workstation. The advantage of diffuse lighting is that

☐ The visual field has very few spots (or glare surfaces) in the visual field, and

☐ The contrasts created by the shape of objects become softer. 2) Use light, matte colors and finishes on walls and ceilings for better reflection of indirect lighting and reduce dark shadows and contrast.

Glare

Probable Risks

The sources of direct light like windows and overhead lights that cause reflected light to show up on the monitor make images more difficult to see, resulting in eyestrain and fatigue.

Feasible Solutions

1) The display screen should be placed at right angles to windows and light sources. The task lightings like the desk lamp should be placed in such a way that the light does not reflect on the screen.

2) You should clean the monitor frequently by wiping with a clean and dry cloth. A layer of dust can add to glare.

3) You can help reduce the glare by using blinds or drapes on windows.

Note: Vertical blinds work best for east/west facing windows and horizontal blinds for north/south facing windows.

4) You can attach glare filters directly to the surface of the monitor to reduce glare. Take care that these filters do not significantly decrease screen visibility. In order to redirect lighting, you can install louvers, or "egg crates" in overhead lights.

5) To reduce glare from overhead lighting, you can use barriers or light diffusers on fixtures.

Probable Risks

The users may suffer from discomfort, annoyance, or loss in visual performance and visibility due to the reflected light from polished surfaces such as keyboards.

Feasible Solutions

You can paint your walls and work surfaces to limit reflection around the screen. Use a medium colored, non-reflective paint. Arrange workstations and lighting to avoid reflected glare on the display screen or surrounding surfaces.

Note: It is noticed that a few number of high-powered lamps will minimize glares than a large number of low powered lamps.

- □ You can slightly tilt down the monitor to prevent it from reflecting overhead light.
- □ The computer monitor can be adjusted for dark characters on a light background. This reduces the reflection compared to the light characters on a dark background.

Chapter 11

Ventilation

Probable Risks

1) If the ventilation system is poorly designed or not functioning properly, the user may experience discomfort. For instance, air conditioners or heaters that directly "dump" air on users are bad for health.

2) Your eyes tend to get dried easily due to the dry air, especially if you are wearing contact lenses.

3) If the air circulation in the room is poor, it can result in stuffy or stagnant conditions.

4) Your comfort and hence the productivity is affected if the temperatures are above or below standard comfort levels.

Feasible Solutions

1) If the air conditioning vents in your workplace are not designed to redirect the flow of air away from the underneath areas of the vents, try not to place desks, chairs, and other office furniture in these areas.

2) In order to redirect and mix airflows from ventilation systems, you can use diffusers or blocks.

3) Try to keep the airflow rates within three and six inches per second (7.5 and 15 centimeters per second). In fact, these airflow rates are barely noticeable or not noticeable at all.

4) The relative humidity of the air should be maintained between 30% and 60%.

5) During hot season, try to maintain the ambient indoor temperature between 68° and 74° F (20° and 23.5° C). During cold season, the recommended temperature is between 73° and 78° F (23° and 26° C).

Probable Risks

The users will have discomfort and several health problems if they are exposed to chemicals, volatile organic compounds (VOCs), ozone, and other particles from computers and their peripherals (say, laser printers).

Feasible Solutions

1) Before purchasing a computer and its components, do investigate about its potential to emit air ventilation diffuser pollutants. The components that are identified to emit pollutants should be placed in well-ventilated areas in your office..

2) You need to ensure sufficient supply of fresh air to maintain proper ventilation in your office room.

3) Before installing the new equipments, you must allow them to "air out" in a well-ventilated area.

Chapter 12

Awkward Postures

Usually, the alignment between the user and the computer components and accessory devices is not proper. This makes it difficult for the user to maintain good postures, such as straight wrists, elbows close to the body, and head straight and in -line with the torso. Let's see a few instances that we face in our everyday life to which causes such misalignment:

1) When your monitor is positioned too high, you tend to tilt your head back, which fatigues the neck and shoulder muscles.

2) If your keyboard tray is too small, you tend to move the mouse to a position of the desk that requires you to reach to perform mouse tasks. This pulls the elbow away from the body and can cause you to support your arm in an elevated position for prolonged hours leading to discomfort and fatigue.

3) If your keyboard is too low, you tend to bend your wrists at extreme angles, which can cause the finger tendons and tendon sheaths to bend around the bones of the wrist. Sitting in such awkward postures irritate or strain the bone-tendon-muscle connections.

4) Muscles when stretched or compressed become inefficient resulting in possible fatigue and overexertion.

5) Postures that are not neutral ones can pull and stretch tendons, blood vessels, and nerves over ligaments or bone thus increasing their chances of becoming pinched and restricted.

6) Tendons and their sheaths can rub on bone and ligaments leading to irritation and fraying. This in turn leads to swelling within confined areas such as the carpal tunnel, which then restricts nerves and blood vessels.

7) The user may also suffer from tingling and numbness of the fingers and hands as well as pain from tendonitis and tenosynovitis (inflammation of a tendon sheath). If the workstation is properly adjusted, it can help the users to minimize awkward postures. It is ideal to place the monitor in front of you at a height where you can look straight ahead and not tilt your head forward or backward. You can keep the items that you access frequently such as keyboards and pointing devices very near to you so that you don't have to strain yourself while reaching out for them every time. You need to adjust and position keyboard trays and chairs so that you don't have to bend your wrists up, down, or to the side. Adjust the chair so as to give good support to your feet and back. If you maintain proper neutral postures, you can work with minimal stress on the musculoskeletal system.

Contact Stress

There are two types of contact stress - internal and external. When a tendon, nerve, or blood vessel is stretched or bent around a bone or tendon, you suffer from internal contact stress. When a part of your body rubs against a component or device in the workstation, like chair seat pan or the desk edge, you are said to be suffering from external contact stress. This may lead to irritation of the nerves or contraction of the blood vessels.

1) The users experience contact stress to their forearms when they rest them on the leading edges of worktables or, if the nerves in the forearm are affected, their fingers and hands may tingle and feel numb, similar to the feeling when they hit their "funny bone".

2) If blood circulation is cut off by contact with the leading edge of a chair, the users are sure to experience pain and numbness in their legs.

3) The forearms and wrists can be affected if the edges of the wrist rests are sharp and hard leading edges.

4) If the wrist is kept bent throughout the jobs like typing which is a repetitive finger motion task, the tendons are sure to get damaged.

You can solve such problems by carefully selecting wrist rests, chairs, and desk surfaces as well as by taking frequent rest and stretch breaks to minimize the amount of contact stress that you may experience. Your workstation should be adjusted in such a way as to maintain neutral wrist postures.

Force

Usually, when we talk about force, it is thought of as a strenuous physical exertion, such as when lifting a heavy weight or pushing a heavy load. In computer parlance, force is totally different from the usual definition. Computer work seldom requires this type of laborious exertion, but there are tasks that require concentrated force that can affect smaller, localized muscle groups.

For instance...

1) Pretend you are using a pointing device that is too sensitive that you find it so difficult to control. There are all chances that your finger and forearm muscles become sore because the muscles of hand and arm must work hard continually to keep the device steady.

2) Pretend your mouse is placed very far from you that you have difficulty reaching for it every time. This time what really happens is that your shoulder and neck muscles become strained as they are continually being used to lift the arm away from your body.

3) Pretend your monitor is kept very high from the recommended height. You tend to tilt your head back to get a clear view of the monitor. This time the muscles of your back can become strained due to continued use.

Normally, when injuries happen, the first point of pain is the muscle. But, the tendon, which attaches the muscle to bone, can also be affected. Localized pain, stiffness, and tenderness are some of the symptoms showing that the muscle or tendon has been exerted beyond its capacity. If you arrange the computer and associated components in your workstation properly and appropriately, so as to maintain neutral postures, you can avoid such problems to a large extend. Select adjustable furniture so that you can minimize the amount of time spent in one posture.

General Controls

Keep in mind the following body postures when you arrange your work components and purchase new equipments:

1) Do not bent or twist your head and neck. Keep them vertical and in-line with the spine.

2) Maintain a straight torso. It should not be twisted, especially when lifting or bending.

3) Whether in standing or sitting postures, keep your torso vertical or within 20 to 30 degrees of vertical.

4) Avoid reaching your elbows frequently to your side, in front, or above your head. Keep them close to your body.

5) Your forearms should be placed approximately parallel to the floor.

6) Do not rotate your forearm repeatedly, especially when your wrist is bent. Try to maintain a neutral forearm posture whenever possible.

7) Your wrists should be kept straight and in-line with your forearms. Do not bent them up or down or to either side.

8) Your thighs should be placed approximately parallel to the floor and your hips slightly higher than your knees.

9) Your feet should be placed firmly on the floor and your legs approximately perpendicular to the floor.

10) Your keyboard and mouse should be placed close together at about the same height to minimize reaching.

11) If you use a fully adjustable chair, it supports your body fully so that you can change your body postures frequently.

12) Your work surface should be height adjustable so that multiple users can sit with their feet firmly on the floor. Do use an adjustable footrest if the work surface is not fully adjustable.

13) All frequently used components such as monitor, keyboard, and mouse should be placed in front of you so that you don't have to turn your head from side to side every time you reach them.

14) Your monitor needs to be placed low enough so its top is not above your horizontal line of sight. This will minimize the need for you to tilt your head backward to see the screen.

15) It is important to provide auxiliary, full-sized, keyboards and monitors if you are using laptops as primary work computers where intensive keyboard use is necessary.

Repetition

Most of the jobs that we do on the computer are highly repetitive in nature. We may perform the same motions repeatedly at a fast pace and with little variation. The recovery time for the muscles and tendons become insufficient when your motions are isolated and repeated frequently for prolonged periods. The risk of injury is more if you combine repetitive tasks with factors such as awkward postures and force.

Computers require little task variation. Old typing activities, such as adding paper or mechanically advancing pages, have been reduced or eliminated. Now, users can stay in their chairs and type/perform mouse work for prolonged hours. A proficient typist can easily perform more than 18,000 keystrokes per hour in such conditions. Such kind of repetitive motions can cause tendon and tendon sheath injuries, especially if the wrist is bent during the activity.

The same is the case while using a pointing device such as a mouse. Here, the risk is greater because the concentration is only on a few fingers of a single hand.

Most of the computer operators usually remain in essentially the same posture for an entire shift. This forces a few isolated muscles to repeatedly activate to accomplish a task such as holding the head up or focusing on a computer screen.

A poorly designed workstation may force the user to repeatedly reach to use a mouse or answer the phone. This can fatigue the muscles of the shoulder and irritate the tendons.

By properly arranging the workstation and its components, you can reduce repetition. Ideally, a mouse that is placed close to the keyboard should minimize repetitive reaching. However, for jobs like data entry operation, even the best-designed workstation cannot eliminate all highly repetitive motions. Hence, it is extremely important to maintain good posture by providing adequate adjustability at the workstation. All hand jobs should be performed with the wrist in a straight, neutral posture to allow the tendons to slide easily without interference. The following work process suggestions may also help reduce repetition.

Task Rotation or Job Enlargement - Doing the same job for prolonged hours in front of the computer is monotonous as well as tiring. If your job involves a variety of other tasks too along with the computer job, manage your time and mix the tasks so that you don't have to strain yourself from doing the same job for long time. Other non-computer tasks such as photocopying, phone work, filing papers, cleaning up, etc. can be done taking short breaks.

Micro Breaks or Rest Pauses – You need to make it a habit to take short rest pauses while doing computer tasks. It is recommended to take short breaks frequently to avoid any kind of stress or strain. You can look at a farther distance, stretch your arms and feet, get up from your chair, or walk for sometime every hour taking a five-minute break. By taking such brief rest pauses, you are giving ample time for your muscles and tendons to recover.

Chapter 13

Musculoskeletal Disorders (MSD)

Msds can range from general aches and pains to more serious problems. Medical practitioners do recommend that all the users who use computers regularly should report signs and symptoms as early as possible to prevent serious injury or permanent damage. The most commonly noticed signs and symptoms of MSD associated with computer use are as follows:

Signs and Symptoms

1) Numbness or a burning sensation in the hand

2) Reduced grip strength in the hand

3) Swelling or stiffness in the joints

4) Pain in wrists, forearms, elbows, neck, or back followed by discomfort

5) Reduced range of motion in the shoulder, neck, or back

6) Dry, itchy, or sore eyes

7) Blurred or double vision

8) Aching or tingling

9) Cramping

10) Loss of color in affected regions

11) Weakness

12) Tension stress headaches and related ailments

These types of problem can be caused by any of the following factors:

- If the user maintains an unnatural or unhealthy posture while using the computer
- If the lower back support is inadequate for the user
- If the user continues to sit in the same position for an extended period of time
- If the set up of the workstation is ergonomically poor.

It should be noticed that all these symptoms might not necessarily lead to an MSD. However, if the user experiences any of the above symptoms, he/she should make an evaluation of their working positions as well as the layout of their workstation.

Prevention Is Better Than Cure...Always

It is always better to take precautions to avoid musculoskeletal disorders than to treat them after you get affected. Some general precautions include:

- Taking regular breaks from working at your computer - a few minutes at least once an hour
- Alternating work tasks like mixing computer tasks with non computer tasks alternately to avoid strain
- Regular stretching to relax your body
- Using comfort equipment such as footrests, wrist/palm rests, and document holders if required
- Keeping the mouse and keyboard at the same level
- Avoiding gripping your mouse too tightly – it is always recommended to hold the mouse lightly and click gently

- Familiarize yourself with keyboard shortcuts for applications you regularly use like Ctrl+S to save and Ctrl+P to print (to avoid overusing the mouse).

As discussed earlier, ensure that your workstation is set up correctly. Normally, it includes the monitor, keyboard, mouse, seating, desk, and where appropriate, footrest (to help you rest your feet flat if they don't reach the floor), wrist rest, and document holder.

The monitor should possess the following features:

- Your monitor should swivel, tilt and elevate - if not use an adjustable stand, books, or blocks to adjust the height
- It should be positioned so the top line of the monitor is not higher than your eyes or not lower than 20° below the horizon of your eyes or field of vision
- Ensure that it is at the same level and near the document holder if you use one
- It should be between 18 to 24 inches away from your face

The keyboard should possess the following features:

- It should be detachable and adjustable (with legs to adjust angle)

- It should allow your forearms to be parallel to the floor without having to raise your elbows
- It should allow your wrists to be in line with your forearms so your wrists need not be flexed up or down
- It should include enough space to rest your wrists or should include a padded detachable wrist rest (or you can use a separate gel wrist rest which should be at least 50 mm deep)

- It should be placed directly in front of the monitor and at the same height as the mouse, track ball, touch pad, or any other pointing device.

The chair should possess the following features:

- It should support the back, and have a vertically adjustable independent back rest that returns to its original position and should have tilt adjustment to support the lower back
- It should allow the user to adjust its height to be adjusted from a sitting position
- It should be adjusted so the back crease of the knee is slightly higher than the pan of the chair (use a suitable footrest, if required)
- It should be supported by a five prong caster base
- Ensure that it has removable and adjustable armrests
- It should also have a contoured seat with breathable fabric and rounded edges to distribute the weight and should be adjustable to allow the seat pan to tilt forward or back

The table/desk should possess the following features:

- Ensure that your table/desk provides ample leg room and is height adjustable (preferably)
- It should have enough room to support the computer equipment and space for documents

- ☐ It should be at least 900 mm deep
- ☐ It should have rounded and blunt corners and edges

Repetitive Strain Injury (RSI)

The work pattern of computer professionals carries a lot of orthopedic disorders. The chief complaint is constant pain in the upper limbs, neck, shoulders, and back. Upper limb disorders (also called RSI, or tenosynovitis) are the most worse as they may rapidly lead to permanent incapacity.

Repetitive strain injury occurs when the movable parts of the limbs are injured. Most of the times, the victims of this injury are computer professionals, musicians, students, and others who have to use their hands regularly in a repetitive manner.

Symptoms

The users experience constant pain in the hands, elbows, shoulders, neck, and the back. Other symptoms are cramps, tingling, and numbness in the hands. The hand movements of the user may become clumsy and the person may find it difficult even to fasten buttons.

Another variant may produce painful symptoms in the upper limbs, but the site may be difficult to locate.

The common diagnoses seen in this group are Carpal Tunnel Syndrome, Tenosynovitis, Bursitis, White Limb, and Shoulder pain. A major cause is strain due to long unbroken periods of work. Ergonomics or the lack of it plays a very important role. Lack of information about the condition leads to neglect by the concerned individuals.

Palliative measures

People concerned should seek medical attention when early symptoms set in. Measures that can be adopted at an individual level include:

Posture: The recommended posture to sit in front of a computer is semi-reclined with the forearms resting in a cradle or on an extension of the keyboard support. There should be ample support for the back. The hands should be free and point in the direction of the forearms. The feet should rest on the ground or feet support. The distance of the monitor should be 18 inches or more and at a slightly lower level than the eye level.

Rest: The user should take short breaks every 15 minutes and slightly long breaks after every hour.

Hydration: Drink adequate fluids to keep the tendons and soft tissues soft.

Shortcuts: Use keyboard shortcuts and less of mouse. Touch the keyboard softly and do not pound at it. The wrist should rest on the table or wrist rest.

Telephone use: Don't cradle the telephone between the face and shoulder while working, as this can lead to neck strain.

Messages: Don't use the computer while conveying messages in person or through the intercom.

No games: Games or surfing at work may increase stress on your hands.

Preventive Measures at the Organizational Level: Organizations that use computers in a big way can also adopt certain preventive measures. These include

- o You need to educate your employees on the importance of adopting a proper posture
- o Ensure that all your employees are using quality ergonomic furniture that will save loss of working hours by guaranteeing full comfort of the employees.
- o Give periodic reminders through lectures and audio-visual presentations by medical professionals on the importance of taking good care of health while using computers.

When symptoms set in, consult an orthopedic surgeon. Do not make the diagnosis yourself. The diagnosis will be made from the history and clinical findings as there will be no changes in X-rays, since the soft tissues are involved. Nerve conduction studies can confirm the diagnosis. In cases detected earlier, attention to ergonomics will restore normalcy.

In cases diagnosed late, orthopedic treatment like injections and even minor surgery may be necessary.

CARPAL TUNNEL SYNDROME

Signs and symptoms:

1) Sore tendons
2) Burning, numb, or rubbery joints, wrist, hand, and shoulder muscles
3) Spasm in a muscle, including back and neck muscles.

Carpal tunnel and any other form of tendonitis or repetitive motion injury can be crippling for computer users and artists. There are even people who can no longer sit at the computer and have to stand or kneel down to get their work done. Even artists find it difficult to use their hands due to this problem.

What should you do?

It is very important that your hand and wrist are in level with each other. There should be no angling up or down of the hand. They should be in the same level when your forearm is horizontal and parallel to the floor, and your upper arm should hang straight down, in a relaxed position. Hence, your keyboard and mouse area should be fairly low, close to your lap. If you find yourself lifting your shoulder, unconsciously, or tilting your wrist to raise your forearm to a comfortable level, your keyboard and mouse are not low enough. You can raise your chair, especially if you remove the center drawer of your desk, and use a footrest to keep your legs in a comfortable, supported position. Don't tense your legs to keep from falling forward -- if you find yourself doing that, your chair is too far from the desk, is tilted forward, or is not giving you good back support. A footrest can help. Make sure you are sitting comfortably upright, with your lower back supported.

It is equally important that your arms and wrists are fully supported on a resilient surface. See to it that your arms are not resting on the sharp edge of a table or shelf! You can use a folded hand towel for padding. It provides a soft surface with an easily adjustable height. Moreover it is very comfortable and inexpensive.

Once you establish a comfortable position for your arms and body, you are not still fully safe. As your keyboard and mouse force you to hold the same position for long periods of time, you have all chances of incurring repetitive motion injury. You can try changing the mouse types every couple of weeks. You can shift from a rolling mouse to a track-ball, from a track-ball to a graphics tablet or other pointing devices. The longer you stick with one, the more repetitive motion injury you will cause. Once a tendon is inflamed it may take months or years to heal because very little blood flows in that area.

EYESTRAIN

Eyestrain is the most common weariness that most computer users all over the world experience. A number of symptoms associated with eyestrain have been experienced and proved worldwide. Let's have a look at some of the symptoms related to vision here:

- ☐ Visual fatigue
- ☐ Blurred or double vision
- ☐ Burning and watering eyes
- ☐ Headaches and frequent changes in prescription glasses

This is now called under the nickname, computer vision syndrome or C.V.S.

American Optometric Association defines, C.V.S as *"A complex of eye and vision problems which are experienced during and related to computer use"*.

There is a basic problem with the prolonged viewing of computer screens. The nature of screen characters and images necessitates subtle but continual refocusing. If one has to regularly switch the attention between a close screen and more distant workspace objects things become more complicated. C.V.S
results from this change in dynamics.

Another cause is that the average person blinks approximately 4 times per minute, far less than the natural rate of 22 blinks per minute. This lower blink rate causes eye moisture to evaporate, resulting in a "dry eye" condition . The symptoms of dry eye are sensations such as itching, burning, blurring, heavy eyelids, fatigue and double vision.

There is no evidence yet that computer work causes permanent eye damage. But the temporary discomfort that may occur can reduce productivity, cause lost work time, and reduce job satisfaction and self-confidence of the user.

In most cases eyestrain results from visual fatigue or glare from bright windows or strong light sources, light reflecting off the display screen, or poor display screen contrast.

Methods to Avoid Eyestrain

- Give ample exercise to the eyes by periodically focusing on objects at varying distances
- Blink the eyes regularly
- Try to keep the air around you moist – For instance, you can use plants, open pans of water or a humidifier (spider plants are said to be particularly good for this and removing chemical vapors from the air)

- Adjust the screen height/seating so that while you are comfortably seated, your eyes are in line with the top of the monitor screen
- Adjust the brightness control on your monitor for comfort. Focusing on the monitor for a long time with full brightness can cause eyestrain.
- Adjust the contrast on your monitor to make the characters distinct from the background
- Adjust the refresh rate of your monitor to stop it flickering
- You need to position monitors in order to avoid glare (e.g. not directly in front of windows)
- Keep your monitor screen clean
- Keep the screen and document holder (if you use one) at the same distance from your eyes
- Try to place the reference materials as close to the screen as possible
- You need to service, repair, or replace monitors that flicker or have insufficient clarity
- Do regular eye testing at least once every 2 years and more frequently if necessary - especially if you are experiencing eye problems related to using display equipment. Specify the distance from your eyes to the monitor to your optician and get information regarding special lenses or the use of bifocals.
- Wear rigid rather than soft contact lens

Summary

In most organizations, computers are an essential tool to get the work done. Though it creates quite a lot of problems, with the proper equipment, ergonomic workstation design, proper techniques and working practices, the risk of problems can be greatly reduced. The law places certain responsibilities firmly with the employer, however, as individuals there are practical measures we all can and should take to avoid harming our health.

Do you have a condition such as computer vision syndrome (CVS), amblyopia (lazy eye), strabismus (turned eye), or a brain injury?

Vision plays a critical role in our learning, working, and recreation. Vision is more than just having 20/20 eyesight. Vision can be defined as the ability to take in information through our eyes and process the information so that it has meaning.

It is very important that our visual system is efficient because two-thirds of all information we receive is visual. About, 75%-90% of classroom learning comes through our visual system. The visual system is composed of 20 visual abilities. Let's have a look at these visual abilities:

- Distance and near acuity: The ability to see clearly at a far distance such as 20 feet, and the ability to see clearly at a near distance such as 16 inches.

- Accommodation: The ability to adjust focus on objects with various distances.

- Binocularity: The ability to use both eyes as a team. Proper eye alignment and coordination is necessary so that the eyes can unite two images into one (fusion), which allows an individual to perceive a single three-dimensional image (depth perception, stereopsis).

☐ Oculomotor skills: The ability to quickly and accurately move our eyes. These skills allow us to move our eyes so we can direct and maintain a steady visual attention on an object (fixation), move our eyes smoothly from point to point as in reading (saccades), and efficiently track a moving object (pursuits).

☐ Peripheral vision: The ability to see or be aware of what is surrounding us (our side vision).

☐ Visual-sensory integration: Once the visual data is gathered, it is processed and combined in the brain with information from hearing (auditory-visual integration), balance (bilateral integration/gross-motor), posture, and movement (eye hand coordination, visual-motor integration).

☐ Visual perceptual skills: The ability to organize and interpret information that is seen and give it meaning is called visual perceptual skills. These information-processing skills include figure-ground, form constancy, spatial relations, visual closure, visual discrimination, visual memory, and visualization.

☐ Figure-ground: The ability to recognize distinct shapes from their background, such as objects in a picture, or letters on a chalkboard   is   called   figure-ground.

- Form constancy: The ability to recognize two objects that have the same shape but different size or position is called form constancy. This ability is needed to tell the difference between "b" and "d", "p" and "q", "m" and "w" are some of these.

- Spatial relations: The ability to judge the relative position of one object to another (directionality) and the internal awareness of the two sides of the body (laterality) is called spatial relations. These skills allow the individual to develop the concepts of right, left, front, back, up, and down. This is needed in reading and mathematics.

- Visual closure: The ability to identify or recognize a symbol or object when the entire object is not visible is called visual closure.

- Visual discrimination: The ability to discriminate between visible likeness and differences in size, shape, pattern, form, position, and color is known as visual discrimination. Such as the ability to distinguish between similar words like "ran" and "run".

- Visual memory: The ability to recall and use visual information from the past is called visual memory.

- Visualization: The ability to create or alter new images in the mind is visualization. It is needed in reading and playing sports.

The basic skills used to perform tasks such as reading and using a computer are these visual abilities. According to the American

Optometric Association, "Among school-age children, vision disorders affect one in every four. While many of these patients have refractive errors (myopia (nearsightedness), hyperopia (farsightedness), and/or astigmatism) commonly treated by compensatory lenses, some have additional problems in the functioning of the vision system that are most appropriately treated with optometric vision therapy". It has been found that about 40% of all Americans have functional vision deficits. Such kinds of vision problems not only affect an individual's ability to perform tasks, but it can also affect his/her self-esteem as well.

Different visual abilities such as distance and near acuity, accommodation (eye focusing), binocularity (eye coordination/eye teaming), oculomotor (eye movement), peripheral vision, and visual perceptual skills such as figure-ground, form constancy, spatial relations, visual closure, visual discrimination, visual memory, and visualization are required when a person does the reading task. People who suffer from Learning Disabilities, Dyslexia, or Attention Deficit Disorder, face yet another obstacle when poor visual abilities are present. Sometimes children who are having visual problems may be mislabeled as Learning Disabled (LD), Dyslexic, Attention Deficit Disorder (ADD), or Attention Deficit Disorder with Hyperactivity (ADHD).

Visual abilities such as visual acuity, accommodation (eye focusing), binocularity (eye coordination/eye teaming), oculomotor skills (eye movement), eye hand coordination, depth perception, peripheral vision, and visualization are all very important skills that are used in sports such as archery, baseball, basketball, football, golf, gymnastics, hockey, racquetball, shooting, skiing, soccer, tennis, and volleyball.

Computer vision syndrome (CVS) is a condition that affects many computer users. Studies show that approximately 70% of computer workers have vision problems. The symptoms of CVS include eyestrain, dry or burning eyes, blurred vision, headaches, double vision, distorted color vision, and neck and backaches. This condition can be due to various factors. One factor is poor visual skills such as accommodative (eye focusing) skills or binocularity (eye coordination/eye teaming) skills. Another factor is the tendency of computer users to stare at monitors for long periods without changing eye focus from time to time. The distance between a computer user and a monitor is another factor. Room lighting, monitor glare, screen color, print color, and print size can also be contributing factors to this condition.

Medical conditions such as amblyopia (lazy eye), strabismus (turned eye), and brain injuries can have a major affect on your vision. Amblyopia causes reduced acuity in the affected eye, poor eye hand coordination, and poor depth perception. Strabismus can cause double vision and poor depth perception. Brain Injuries, such as Traumatic Brain Injury (TBI), Mild Acquired Brain Injury, Mild Closed Head injury, Post-Concussive Syndrome, Cervical Trauma Syndrome, Post Traumatic Vision Syndrome, Stroke, Cerebral Palsy, and Cerebral Vascular Accident, can cause a reduced visual field (reduced peripheral vision), double vision, and other vision problems.

Symptoms of a Vision Problem

- Reading and/or using a computer causes eyes to tear, itch, or hurt.
- Jerky eye movements.
- Eyes that cross or turn in or out.
- Squinting, eye rubbing, or excessive blinking.
- Blurred vision.
- Light sensitivity after reading.
- Double vision.
- Headaches, dizziness, nausea, or fatigues easily after reading.
- Head tilting, closing or blocking one eye when reading.
- Skips lines or loses place when reading.
- Difficulty tracking moving objects.
- Misaligning letters or numbers.
- Unusual posture or moving head closely to see book or paper.
- Avoidance of near work such as reading.
- While reading, you feel that words, letters, or lines run together or jump around.
- Difficulty concentrating or comprehending reading material.
- Persistent reversals of numbers, letters, or words after second grade.
- Writes crooked or poorly spaced.
- Poor eye hand coordination.
- Inconsistent or poor sports performance.

Optometric Vision Therapy

Vision therapy, an optometric specialty treatment, has been clinically shown to be an effective treatment for accommodative disorders (non-presbyopic eye focusing problems), binocular dysfunction (inefficient eye teaming), ocular motility dysfunctions (eye movement disorders), strabismus (turned eye), amblyopia (lazy eye), and perceptual-motor dysfunction. Many vision disorders can be treated with corrective lenses such as glasses or contacts, while other disorders may be most effectively treated with optometric vision therapy or with a combination of the two.

Visual skills such as accommodation (eye focusing), binocularity (eye coordination/eye teaming), oculomotor (eye movement skills), and eye hand coordination are neuro-muscular abilities. These visual skills are controlled by the muscles inside and outside the eye and are networked with the brain. Neuro-muscular abilities are learned and are developmental in nature. There is a general misconception that weak visual skills will go away with time. But, studies show that it has to be treated properly. Binocularity (eye coordination/eye teaming), oculomotor (eye movement skills), and eye hand coordination can be retrained to perform more efficiently at almost any age. Accommodation (eye focusing) can be improved until the person's age is 40.

Optometric vision therapy is a set of procedures that are individualized and prescribed by an optometrist to teach a patient how to improve a weak or nonexistent visual skill or processing skill through the use of lenses, prisms, special computer programs, and other treatment techniques. This is a treatment to improve a specific vision disorder; it is not a treatment for dyslexia, learning disabilities, or attention deficit disorder.

Weak visual and processing skills reduce the individual's ability to quickly and accurately comprehend the reading material. Reading and learning become easier after the skills are improved through the treatment of vision therapy.

The visual abilities, which are needed in sports, can be trained through vision therapy to reach their maximum potential. Computer vision syndrome (CVS) may be improved by vision therapy, prescription glasses, or modifications to the workstation. Users can seek the help of an optometrist to determine if their accommodative (eye focusing) or binocularity (eye coordination/eye teaming) skills are adequate.

Research studies have shown that children and adults with amblyopia (lazy eye) and strabismus (turned eye) may be able to improve their visual performance and function through vision therapy. For many years, it was thought that amblyopia (lazy eye) and strabismus (turned eye) was only amenable to treatment during the "critical period". This is the period up to age seven or eight years. However, recent research has demonstrated that effective treatment can occur at any age, but the length of the treatment period increases dramatically, if this condition has existed for a prolonged time prior to treatment.

The prognosis for strabismus can vary from very poor to excellent depending on the type of deviation, type and number of visual adaptations (suppression, abnormal retinal correspondence, or amblyopia), duration of condition, and prior interventions. A study by Dr. Gary Etting, O.D., F.C.O.V.D. in 1978 showed that 57% of patients with constant esotropia and 82% with constant exotropia had a functional and cosmetic cure with vision therapy. The cure rate was 100% for patients with intermittent esotropia and 85% for patients with intermittent exotropia. Individuals with mild or no amblyopia, normal retinal correspondence, some depth perception, and a deviation that remains essentially the same in all positions of gaze will have a better prognosis than someone who does not. If you want to find out whether this would be an effective treatment for you, do consult an optometrist who specializes in vision therapy.

People suffering from brain injuries and certain types of vision problems can benefit a lot from vision therapy. The Neuro-Optometric Rehabilitation Association International, Inc. (NORA) provides more information about various treatment options available for those with vision problems and brain injuries.

Vision therapy is a very old technique. Physicians in the mid-1800s originally introduced many of the techniques that are used today. Modern Optometric Vision Therapy was pioneered in the United States in 1928 by optometrist A. M. Skeffington. Throughout the years, vision therapy has been called various names such as visual training, orthoptics, or eye exercises.

A few insurance companies cover optometric vision therapy, if it is addressing a condition that is classified as a disease such as convergence insufficiency. Vision therapy falls under the area of Major Medical. Insurance companies classify vision therapy as "Orthoptics" with a CPT (procedure) code of 92065. If this treatment procedure is covered, the percentage of coverage and the number of sessions covered can vary greatly. Vision therapy is not generally covered by vision care plans that simply cover eye examinations, eyeglasses, or contact lenses.

Other Computer Hazards

GAS from COMPUTERS and other sources

Computers give off different types of gasses. Some people are highly sensitive to these gasses. One source of this 'gas' is the plastic components; most plastics are unstable and break down naturally over time, especially when exposed to ultraviolet light and sunlight. (That's the reason why they turn yellow and brittle.) The gasses given off by this breakdown are called **'out-gassing'** and only occur in small amounts. But when the equipment is new, the out-gassing is much greater and noticeable even to people who aren't particularly sensitive. This is similar to the smell that we get when we enter a new car. That smell is out-gassing from the vinyl, plastic carpet and hard plastic interiors, as well as the wiring. A new computer has a similar smell.

People who have been sensitized (by previous exposure to plastic solvents) may react to even small amounts of this gas by getting headaches, dizziness, and respiratory problems, etc. Chips and printed circuits use mercury-based compounds that give off a gas when current flows through them. The solution is to work in a room with good ventilation.

Other office materials: New office furnishings are also nasty - chipboard uses phenolic resins and formaldehydes; carpeting (especially foam padding), paint and fabrics give off obnoxious chemicals when new. So you need to open every window you can for as many days as you can. The solvents in whiteout, rubber cement thinner and permanent magic marker (like Sharpies) cause "damage to the central and peripheral nervous system." Toluene, xylol, xylene, benzine, n-hezane, etc. are truly toxic. Contact the manufacturers for more info. It has be experienced that latex causes serious reactions in hospitals.

LASER PRINTERS and breathing problems

Laser printers emit a lot of toner dust, which contains carbon and solvents, and quite a few people are sensitive to it. You can smell it when the printer is on, and especially on freshly printed-paper. You may notice wheeziness, coughing, sneezing, etc. People working at copy centers and service bureaus suffer from headaches, and suspect the toner dust. NCR paper ('carbonless' paper) can also cause wheeziness. Good ventilation, drawing air away from the operator would help reduce such reactions.

Good ventilation in a commercial or home office is sometimes hard to achieve, especially in sealed buildings. You can try going outdoors and breathing deeply for 10 minutes every hour or so.

MONITORS and HEADACHES

Radiation is a well-known problem. More radiation is emitted by the back of the monitor than the screen, so you, your co-workers and family members should never sit close to the back of your computer.

Another hazard is the headache produced by the almost invisible 'flicker' of the monitor as the image on screen is refreshed. The solution is to increase the refresh rate of the monitor to at least 75hz. Your monitor driver or control panel should offer you a choice of refresh rates. To find out if your monitor is flickering, pay attention only to the view in your peripheral vision. If you see a faint flicker, or find yourself getting frequent headaches, increase your refresh rate, reduce the contrast on screen, sit further from the screen, and increase the ambient lighting around your workstation.

Standard fluorescent lights also flicker and can cause headaches or dizziness. If you can, use reflected light from halogens or daylight-spectrum fluorescents - shine the light onto the ceiling or wall, never toward your eyes. Best of all is reflected daylight, but don't allow glare on the screen.

The way you position your head is also important. Your monitor should be placed below the level of your head, and tilted slightly upward, so your gaze is slightly downward, putting your neck in a more natural, relaxed position.

Note: NEVER work past the point of discomfort. Stretch out for ten minutes - right now - save your hands, arms, back and maybe your career.

Chemicals From Computers

Studies have shown that computers themselves are housing some of the most dangerous chemicals on earth. Let's have a look at a few of them and their effects on mankind.

Lead

Lead is one of the few natural substances that have no use in the human body. At even very low levels, Lead has been shown to cause health problems. The difficulty with Lead is that once it is mined from the earth, there is no known way to destroy or make it harmless.

Lead can damages the central and peripheral nervous systems, blood system and kidneys in humans. Lead accumulates in the environment and has effects on plants, animals and microorganisms.

Consumer electronics constitute 40% of lead found in landfills and scrap yards. An average computer uses 4 pounds of Lead, i.e., 6.2% of the total weight of the PC. The recyclable efficiency of Lead is a low 5%.

The main uses of Lead in Consumer Electronics are for soldering of PCBs and other electronic components as well as Glass panels in computer monitors (cathode ray tubes).

As computers become obsolete, more and more lead gets accumulated which is harmful to our health.

Cadmium

Cadmium is an extremely toxic metal. It has a possible risk of irremediable effects on human health. Cadmium and cadmium compounds amass in the human body, in particular in kidneys. Cadmium is absorbed mainly through respiration but also enters as food. Due to its long half-life period (30 years), cadmium can easily be accumulated in amounts that cause symptoms of poisoning. Cadmium shows a danger of cumulative effects in the environment due to its acute and chronic toxicity.

In electrical and electronic equipment, cadmium occurs in certain components such as SMD, chip resistors, infrared detectors and semiconductors. Older types of cathode ray tubes contain cadmium. Moreover, cadmium is used as a plastic stabilizer. It is also used in Batteries, PWBs, etc.

As computers become obsolete, more and more cadmium gets accumulated which is harmful to our health.

Mercury

Mercury is a powerful poison. Published research has shown that mercury, even in small amounts, is more toxic than lead, cadmium and even arsenic! It is estimated that 22 % of the yearly world consumption of mercury is used in electrical and electronic equipment. It is used in mobile phones, Batteries, PWBs. Although mercury is just 0.0022% of the total weight of the computer, it is still a health hazard. As computers become obsolete, more and more mercury gets accumulated which is harmful to our health.

Other hazardous metals used in electronics are: **Arsenic** (0.0013%), **Barium** (0.0315%), **Selenium** (0.0016%), **Silver** (0.0189%).

Note: These alarming statistics have been revealed to make every one aware of the environmental and health hazards of computers.

Electromagnetic radiation and computer use

The biggest risk to life from computers is electricity. Electric shock from mains voltage is often fatal. Ensure that cables are inserted correctly and are checked regularly. Computers and associated equipment do produce very small electromagnetic fields. There is no evidence that there is any hazard from these fields. There is no risk to unborn children in computer workers who are pregnant.

Work with display screen equipment and computers:

  does not damage eyesight
  does not affect pregnant women or their unborn children

does not cause cancer

Legislation

The Health and Safety (Display Screen Equipment) Regulations 1992 set out the approach that employers have to take with staffs who use computers and display screen equipment as a part of their jobs. The employer must arrange an assessment that covers many of the points mentioned above. If the employer decides that an individual is a "user", the "user" must be offered an eyesight test. If glasses are required to use display screen equipment (and only display screen equipment) the employer must provide corrective lenses. The number of computers in the workplace has increased rapidly over the last few years and it's now almost the norm for most staff in voluntary organizations to be exposed to computer usage.

The Health and Safety at Work Act now lays down legal standards for computer equipment and requires employers to take steps to minimize risks for all workers. Workers have received substantial damages for injuries caused through use of computers where the employer could have foreseen the risk but did nothing about it.

The main regulations covering the use of computer equipment include:

- Health & Safety (Display Screen Equipment) Regulations 1992
- Management of Health & Safety at work Regulations 1992
- Provision and Use of Work Equipment Regulations 1992
- Workplace (Health, Safety and Welfare) Regulations 1992

Improving health and safety practice should be taken seriously although it need not take much time or expense. Measures employers should take include:

- Understanding the law - make sure someone in the organization has a health and safety brief covering all areas and not just computers
- Being aware of the health risks - the government officially recognizes some of the risks although there are some gray areas you'll need to make up your own mind about

- Assessing the risks - using procedures set out in the law - be systematic and get help if you need it. Get a health and safety audit done by a competent organization if necessary
- Taking steps to minimize the risks - this may only involve taking simple measures
- Training all users to recognize the risks - if people aren't aware of the dangers, they can't take adequate precautions to protect their health
- Taking users views seriously - if users feel there is something wrong, there often is something wrong.

Dragon Naturally Speaking

Dragon Naturally Speaking ® Preferred is the most accurate speech recognition product developed by Scan Soft Solutions Provider. The manufacturers claim that this product delivers up to 99% accuracy.

You can replace slow and painful typing with the simplicity of using your voice to turn speech into text at up to 160 words per minute. You can create e-mail, instant messages, documents, and spreadsheets more than three times faster than typing – simply by speaking. Plus, you can use your voice to control your PC. You can start programs, use menus and surf the Web all by voice. This revolutionary product gives you everything you need to get started in minutes – including a free high quality headset microphone with noise canceling technology.

By using this particular product, you can be faster, and have more fun, as you create letters, reports, and e-mail, all by speaking. By talking and doing nothing else, you can surf the Web, open and close applications, even control your mouse and the entire desktop.

Chapter 14

4 Steps to Setting Up Your Computer Workstation

STEP 1: Your Chair

- [ ] The hips should be pushed as far back as possible against the chair.

- [ ] The seat height should be adjusted so that the feet stay flat on the floor and the knees are equal to or slightly lower than the hips.

- [ ] The back of the chair need to be adjusted to a 100°-110° reclined angle. The user should ensure that the upper and lower back is supported. Inflatable cushions or small pillows can be used, if required. Frequent position changes can be made in chairs with active back mechanism.

- [ ] The armrest (if present) can be adjusted to relax the shoulders. If armrests are uncomfortable, immediately remove them.

STEP 2: Your Keyboard

An articulating keyboard tray can provide optimal positioning of input devices. Nevertheless, the important functions of a keyboard tray should be to accommodate the mouse, enable leg clearance, and have an adjustable height and tilt mechanism. The tray should not push the user too far away from other work materials, such as telephone.

- [ ] The user should pull himself/herself close to the keyboard.

- The keyboard should be positioned directly in front of the user's body.
- The user should decide which part of the keyboard he will be using frequently and hence readjust the keyboard so that section is centered with the body.
- The keyboard height needs to be adjusted so that the shoulders are relaxed, elbows are in a slightly open position (100° to 110°), and the wrists and hands are straight.
- The tilt of the keyboard is dependent upon the sitting position of the user. Use the keyboard tray mechanism, or keyboard feet, to adjust the tilt. While sitting in a forward or upright position, the user should try to tilt the keyboard away from him at a negative angle. If the user is reclined, a slight positive tilt will help maintain a straight wrist position.
- Wrist rests are excellent in helping to maintain neutral postures and pad hard surfaces. However, the wrist rest should only be used to rest the palms of the hands between keystrokes. It is not recommended to rest the palms on the wrist rest while typing. Avoid using excessively wide wrist rests, or wrist rests that are higher than the space bar of your keyboard because it might cause strain.
- Place the pointer as close as possible to the keyboard. Placing it on a slightly inclined surface, or using it on a mouse bridge placed over the 10-keypad, can help to bring it closer.

If you do not have a fully adjustable keyboard tray, you may need to adjust your workstation height, the height of your chair, or use a seat cushion to get in a comfortable position. Remember to use a footrest if your feet hang down.

STEP 3: Monitor, Document, and Telephone

If the screen and source documents are not positioned correctly, it may force the user to work in awkward postures. These need to be adjusted so that your neck is in a neutral, relaxed position. Try the following:

- Place the monitor directly in front of you, above your keyboard.
- Position the top of the monitor approximately 2-3" above seated eye level. (If you wear bifocals, lower the monitor to a comfortable reading level.)
- The distance from the screen should be at least an arm's length away and then the distance from your vision is to be adjusted.
- Reduce glare by careful positioning of the screen.
    - Place screen at right angles to windows
    - Adjust curtains or blinds as needed
    - Adjust the vertical screen angle and screen controls to minimize glare from overhead lights
    - Other techniques to reduce glare include use of optical glass glare filters, light filters, or secondary task lights
- Position source documents directly in front of you, between the monitor and the keyboard, using an in-line copy stand. If the space is not enough, place source documents on a document holder positioned adjacent to the monitor.
- Place your telephone within easy reach. Telephone stands or arms can help.
- Use headsets and speakerphone to eliminate cradling the handset.

Chapter 15

Exercises and Breaks

Now, your computer workstation is set up correctly. The next step is to use good work habits. Even if the work environment is absolutely suiting all your requirements and comfort levels, it may still lead to unwanted stresses and strains if good habit is not cultivated. Prolonged, static postures will inhibit blood circulation and take a toll on your body. Try the following:

- Take short 1-2 minute stretch breaks every 20-30 minutes. After each hour of work, take a break or change tasks for at least 5-10 minutes. Always try to get away from your computer during lunch breaks.

- Avoid eye fatigue by resting and refocusing your eyes periodically. Look away from the monitor and focus on something in the distance.

- Rest your eyes by covering them with your palms for 10-15 seconds.

- Use correct posture when working. Keep moving as much as possible.

Some Exercises for Computer Users

"A healthy mind in a healthy body" – this saying is true even for computer users. While working on the computer, your body is at rest and gets typically no exercise. Computer users tend to go out of shape and gain weight apart from the other health problems discussed throughout this book. In the long run, these lead to all kinds of ailments. Why does this happen? Because you become so engrossed in your work that you forget how long you have been sitting in front of the machine! And most badly, you don't get time for workouts in the mornings or evenings due to the tight work schedule.

We have time for anything and everything, but when it comes to workouts, we hardly have time. Let's have a look at some common and refreshing exercises that keeps you fit all day long. These can be done even at your work place during your micro breaks and short breaks.

- **Eyes:**

To the sides: Focus both eyes to your sides, together. Do so to the left and right sides alternately five times each, without turning your neck or head.

Up and down: Similarly, do so to top and bottom five times each alternately. Ensure that your head and neck are steady and are not moving while you move your eyes.

Rotation: Now, rotate your eyes as to form a circle, both eyes focusing together at each point, five times in the clockwise direction and five times in the anticlockwise direction. This exercise can be done at your own comfortable pace.

Neck:

To the sides: Breath in, turn your neck to your right side and bring back to the normal position while you breathe out. This is done five times each to both right and left sides alternately.

Up and down: Similarly, breathe in and tilt your neck up so as to look at the roof. Now, bent down so that your chin touches your body while you breathe out. This is done alternately up and down five times each at your own pace.

Rotation: Now, rotate your neck as to form a circle while you breath normally. While you rotate, your head should be bent down first taking it to one shoulder, then bending back, now touching the other shoulder, and then coming to the initial position. This is done five times in the clockwise direction and five times in the anticlockwise direction. Never overstrain yourself while you do this exercise. The number of times can be reduced according to your convenience and health.

Wrist Rotation: Stretch both arms straight to the front with closed fists. Rotate both the fists together ten times in the clockwise direction and ten times in the anticlockwise direction. Do ensure that only your fists are rotating and the rest of your arms are stationery.

Elbow Rotation: Bend your hands towards the front and hold your shoulders with your palms. Now, rotate your elbows ten times in the clockwise and ten times in the anticlockwise direction.

Whole hands, small circles: Stretch both hands to the sides holding your palms straight up perpendicular to the hands. Now, make small circles with both palms ten times in the clockwise and ten times in the anticlockwise direction. Note that the smaller the circle, the better relaxation to your hands. This is an excellent exercise for those who have to sit in front of the computer for very long hours.

Whole hands, big circles: Stretch your hands to the sides. Make big circles (as big as possible) with both the hands ten times in the clockwise and ten times in the anticlockwise direction. The number of times can be increased gradually as this becomes less strenuous. All these exercises can be done while you relax in your workstation seat. If you prefer doing them at home or in standing postures, you can stand in the 'attention' posture.

Back

Backward: Stand straight in the attention posture. Breath in while you bends back and come back to the normal position while you breathe out. While you bend back, try to bend as much as possible, but without straining your back. Try to do this ten times.

Forward: Stand straight in the attention posture. Raise both hands up while you breath in and come down to touch your toes without bending your knees while you breath out. You might not be able to do it with perfection in the initial days, but can improve gradually day by day. Don't try to touch your toes in the beginning as it might hurt your back. Most users tend to increase their waist length on prolonged use with computers. This is the apt exercise for such people. So be in shape while you work on your PC. You can start off this exercise with five numbers gradually increasing to ten in the first week, fifteen in the second and third weeks, and can go till thirty-five daily if your back permits.

Shoulders: Use a large bath towel and grasp it at opposite corners. Sling it across the shoulder of tightness and bring both ends across to the opposite hip or waist. With the arm on that side pull gently downward and then release slowly.

Apart from these exercises, you can go for jogging, brisk walking, aerobics, swimming, outdoor games etc. to be in good shape and improve your stamina. Remember that you don't get much exercise the whole day when you are in front of your computer. So, sacrifice your one-hour in the mornings or evening for your healthy body to have a healthy mind.

Conclusion

So that is all about it. You know everything that is to be known and the ball is now well and truly in your courts. Living carelessly is the easiest thing to do, but could be the most dangerous thing too. On the other hand if you take some precaution, it can be the foundation for a healthy living, later in your life. Remember that all the computer related hazards are not going to hamper your life in a very short span of time. But it may take years to show the symptoms. As I said earlier, prevention is better than cure. So, why wait any more. It's time to apply the principles explained in the book.

Please see the next page for our recommended computer resources.

Recommended Resources

1) Anti Virus Program. MicroAntiVirus 2006 is the world's most trusted antivirus solution. It protects email, instant messages, and other files by automatically removing viruses.

2) Anti-Virus Solution. Great software, great members area. Secure, protect and clean your pc.

3) High Paying Virus & Spyware Removal Svc. Using Totally Free Software. Become A Professional With Expert Support.

4) Noadware.net - Spyware/Adware Remover. Don't let people invade your privacy and slow down your PC! Try NoAdware for FREE and see for yourself if your PC is infected!

5) Scan And Fix Errors In Windows Registry. Error Nuker - Scan your Pc for Free to Check for Windows Registry Errors

6) XoftSpySe - #1 Converting Anti-Spyware. XoftSpy detects Spyware, Adware, and other Parasites. Free scan!

7) AdwareAlert.com - Are there unseen Trojans, dialers or worms lurking on your computer?

8) SpyWare Detection & Removal Software! Over 8 million people worldwide use nuker to protect their pc. You can try it yourself today absolutely free!

9) New: The Official Spyware Remover! Scan your computer for hidden adware and spyware. Remove them permanently.

www.ingramcontent.com/pod-product-compliance
Lightning Source LLC
Chambersburg PA
CBHW080427060326
40689CB00019B/4406